helping teens who cut

helping teens who cut

Michael Hollander, PhD

THE GUILFORD PRESS
New York   London

© 2008 The Guilford Press
A Division of Guilford Publications, Inc.
72 Spring Street, New York, NY 10012
www.guilford.com

The information in this volume is not intended as a substitute for consultation with health care professionals. Each individual's health concerns should be evaluated by a qualified professional.

Printed in the United States of America

This book is printed on acid-free paper.

Last digit is print number: 9   8   7   6   5   4   3   2   1

Library of Congress Cataloging-in-Publication Data

Hollander, Michael.
    Helping teens who cut : understanding and ending self-injury /
by Michael Hollander.
        p.   cm.
    Includes bibliographical references and index.
    ISBN: 978-1-59385-426-3 (pbk. : alk. paper)
    ISBN: 978-1-59385-705-9 (hardcover : alk. paper)
    1. Self-mutilation in adolescence—Popular works.   I. Title.
    RJ506.S44H635 2008
    618.92′8582—dc22
                                                2008002171

contents

preface

My interest in kids who self-injure was sparked by a conversation I over-heard between two adolescent girls at a hospital and school for troubled kids. I was in my first year of postdoctoral training, and what I heard made me think they were just striking a pose: They were sharing with each other the benefits of self-injury. Speaking with a kind of secret excitement, they told of how burning themselves actually made them feel better and more alive. As I spoke with supervisors and colleagues, my eyes were opened to this phenomenon, and I realized that the girls had indeed been serious. Soon afterward, I began to seek out patients who deliberately self-harmed. Much of what I know about self-injury I learned from my young patients.

Without exception, the parents of these patients were frightened, confused, and worried that they had somehow failed their children. Kids who deliberately hurt themselves need specialized treatment and, in some ways, specialized parenting. Since I am a parent myself, I know that parenting is a challenge even under the best of circumstances. "Once you get on that bus, you can never get off"—these were my mother's words of wisdom to me when my wife and I were about to have our first child, and she was right. While she certainly captured the idea of child rearing as a long-term ride, I didn't fully anticipate the bumpy roads, the storms we would have to drive through, or the occasional breakdowns.

Raising children is very hard work. While each developmental stage presents its own difficulties, adolescence is certainly one of the hardest for parents to negotiate. The journey becomes especially tortuous if our children have emotional difficulties. It's all too easy to get lost ourselves in the emotional storms and breakdowns that overwhelm our kids. Our own understandable worry about our children's emotional states sometimes makes clear thinking impossible. To complicate matters, our health care system sometimes appears designed to prevent our children from getting the help they need to move forward. I hope the following chapters will make your journey progress a little more smoothly.

I have confidence that with a better understanding of self-injury and some new tools to address the problem, your life will get a little easier. My confidence arises from the program data that we routinely collect from kids and parents who have attended our program at Two Brattle Center and from the many conversations that I have had over the years with parents who have tried these techniques. If you learn these skills and begin to use them, you will be more effective with your children.

I have raised one adolescent and am in the process of raising another. I know how challenging this can be. My wife, who is a clinical social worker, and I routinely use the skills outlined in this book both to be useful to our child and to keep ourselves going in the right direction. That's what I hope this book will do for you—send you in the right direction, by giving you some effective tools that make a tough job a bit easier.

acknowledgments

It is impossible to acknowledge all the people who have influenced my clinical thinking over the last 30 years. I have been extremely fortunate to have had the chance to be trained at and then affiliated with McLean Hospital. I would like to acknowledge three master teachers: Richard Bonier, PhD, Edward Shapiro, MD, and Shervert Frazier, MD. These three teachers, each of whom had a very different way of approaching psychological treatment, shaped my clinical work. The time I spent at the Adolescent Day Service and the Adolescent and Family Treatment Unit helped me understand what adolescents need and how their struggles affect their parents, and vice versa. I am deeply grateful for what they were able to teach me.

My acknowledgments and thanks to Cynthia Kaplan, friend and colleague at the McLean Hospital Acute Residential Treatment Program. Her clarity of thought, humor, and support have been invaluable to me over the years.

I want to thank Blaise Aquirre for reviewing the manuscript and making helpful suggestions regarding the use of medications.

Joan Wheelis's vision for treatment has been a major influence in my work and in the writing of this book. I am grateful to her for pushing me to learn dialectical behavior therapy (DBT) and for providing me the opportunity to develop an adolescent DBT program at Two Brattle Center.

I want to thank Shari Manning, PhD, for her help in making sure the chapters about DBT were accurate, precise, and clear.

I am deeply grateful to Mathew Nock, PhD, and Tara Deliberto at Harvard University for their willingness to keep me up to date on the research pertaining to adolescent self-injury.

No one has done more than Marsha Linehan to dramatically expand my clinical thinking. Her rigorous adherence to the science of psychotherapy helped me challenge my beliefs about the process of change, while at the same time her compassion and kindness with patients earned my admiration and respect.

My developmental editor at The Guilford Press, Chris Benton, helped shape this book at every turn. I am immensely grateful to her for sifting the chaff from my thoughts to identify what I was trying to say. Her support, good humor, and keen insight were invaluable to me throughout the writing process.

I want to thank Kitty Moore, Executive Editor at Guilford, for taking a chance on a first-time author, and for keeping me in the game with her irreverence and perspicacity.

Thanks to my daughter, Kate, a writer, for looking over the beginning drafts and for her invaluable cheerleading and commiseration. Thanks also to my son, Sam, for his excellent ear for dialogue and for keeping me humble.

I have the good luck to be married to a thoughtful and skilled clinician, Janna Hobbs, who was truly a partner in the writing of this book. I am grateful to her both for her willingness to sacrifice her time to help me think through the ideas in this book and for providing me with the kind of feedback that sharpened my thinking. Her patience and loving support were a critical part of this process.

INTRODUCTION

kids who deliberately hurt themselves

In more than 30 years as a psychologist, I have helped hundreds of teens with all manner of problems. And I have seen that nothing causes parents as much anguish as kids who deliberately cut, scratch, burn, or hurt themselves in some other fashion. Parents find their children's self-injury to be one of the most painful experiences they have ever had, and one of the most confusing. If you find yourself in this situation, it's only natural for you to be frightened, sad, and sometimes angry. Whatever you try to do to help your child may seem only to make the situation worse. And your frustration may have created tension between you and the child's other parent, who might have very different ideas about how to manage the problem.

My intention in these pages is to clear up the confusion surrounding self-injury, to explain how it can be successfully treated with an intense, short-term program, and to show you what you can do to help. This is not a book about becoming the perfect parent or doing everything right—there's no such thing. No matter how hard we try, we can't always provide our children with what they need, whether it be discipline, empathy, validation, or guidance. We fail because our timing is off, or we misread a situation, or we're tired or angry. We fail because the world has changed so much from when we were young, or because we didn't get what we needed from our own parents, so we just don't know how.

Children, especially emotionally sensitive ones, have a way of bringing our parental weak spots to the surface. I would like you to read this book with compassion for yourself as well as your child. Self-injury is a complicated problem with a multitude of causes. The first thing I want to tell you is, Do not blame yourself. You will probably be able to help your son or daughter the most if you don't try to be perfect and instead focus on staying open to learning from your mistakes. Don't underestimate your strengths. You may need to do things somewhat differently from other parents, but you can learn the skills to be the parent your child needs.

Getting your child professional help will be an important component of what you need to do. In this book I want to introduce you to a relatively new therapy, dialectical behavior therapy (DBT), that has been shown to be effective in helping kids to stop hurting themselves. While it is impossible to predict how long any particular treatment will take, DBT seems to be the shortest and most effective route to wellness. While DBT is not a miracle cure, I've seen kids reduce self-injury in 3 to 6 months. Keep in mind that any therapy is a process of a few steps forward and a step back. It is not a smooth upward course. I also want to offer some tips about how you can be helpful as a parent and how to take care of yourself so you're able to tolerate what can be a very bumpy and uncomfortable ride. I hope by the time you finish this book, you will have a clearer understanding of self-injury and will be armed with the tools to help get your child back on track.

The second thing I want you to understand is that your child is self-injuring because it calms him or her—at least that's true for the vast majority. To us, that's a terrible solution. To your child, it's one that works. We don't know why it works—probably because of some combination of biological and psychological factors we don't fully understand. One of the main purposes of DBT is to help adolescents find other ways to calm and soothe themselves.

Rest assured that you're not alone on this journey. Most self-injury begins in early adolescence, around 13 or 14, and affects an estimated 9% of the teenage population. Let me share with you some brief moments in therapy with two adolescents who self-injure. You will probably find something of your own son or daughter in their responses.

SARA: "IT CALMS ME DOWN"

Sara, age 15, and her parents entered my office for their first consultation. Sara was neatly dressed, had an easy manner, and appeared quite comfortable in this situation. Her father had called earlier and requested the consultation on the advice of Sara's therapist. In the phone call he reported that the therapist wasn't sure they were making any real progress. Her father also said he thought Sara had a good relationship with her therapist, and that Sara said she liked to meet with him but was still cutting. Sara's dad went on to reassure me that the cutting was superficial and never required medical attention. Sara, her father related, was a good student who had many friends but often doubted her own abilities.

Very soon into the visit it was clear that Sara was a bright and personable young woman. She told me that she had been cutting herself since middle school and that she engaged in the behavior two to three times a week, sometimes less—and in times of stress more frequently. When I asked her what she meant by "stress," she described feeling emotionally overwhelmed, like she wanted to "jump out of her skin." When I asked when her parents learned of her behavior, Sara's mom said she had learned of it only 8 months ago, when the school nurse called and told her she had noticed superficial cuts on Sara's shoulders. A cloud of sadness swept across Sara's face, and tears begin to well in her eyes. Right at this moment Sara's dad quickly asserted that as soon as this came to their attention, they found a therapist and set up an appointment for Sara.

I turned to Sara and asked her about her work with her therapist. She told me that she liked him very much and found him very easy to talk to. I asked what kind of things she and her therapist spoke about. "All kinds of stuff," she said, "like school stuff and friend issues."

"Do you speak about your cutting?" I asked.

"No, not very often," she replied, "but I know the doctor doesn't want me to do it. We're trying to understand why I do it—you know, to figure out what it means."

I asked Sara if she felt a sense of relief from stress after she cuts. She replied that she does feel better after she injures herself: "It calms me down." I asked her if she wants to stop cutting, and she assured me that she did.

"Why?" I asked.

She knows it's unhealthy, Sara said, that it worries her parents, and that she doesn't want scars on her body. I told her that while these are very good reasons to stop cutting, in my experience they rarely have been sufficient for someone to stop. I asked her in more detail about the experience of being emotionally overwhelmed. She described feeling "sort of crazy on the inside, like I'm about to get out of control." She let on that cutting had been the only thing that had helped her calm down in these situations.

"How long does the relief last?" I inquired. "And what happens when the relief is gone?"

"It depends," she replied. "Sometimes it lasts a few days and sometimes only a couple of minutes. Afterward I feel kind of guilty. I used to tell myself I won't ever do it again, but I don't do that anymore. I know when I get into that state I don't have any control over myself."

"So cutting really works at helping you manage powerful emotions. It is a simple, relatively easy thing to do. Are you sure you want to stop?" I asked. "Suppose I could convince your parents not to worry about the cutting and reassure you that in the future cosmetic surgery will probably take care of the scars? Would you still want to stop?"

A faint smile appeared on Sara's face as she said, "No. In fact, I really don't want to stop."

Sara's admission that she was not so sure she wanted to stop cutting clearly surprised her parents. It's often the case, however, that adolescents who self-injure have come to realize how effectively the behavior helps them to soothe themselves. It's not at all unusual for them to have mixed feelings about giving it up.

Sara's story highlights two important themes. First, *self-injury usually serves to help kids calm down from an intense emotional state*. Second, *sometimes even good therapists, the kind who really know how to relate to teenagers and are helpful in most situations, can miss the boat on self-injury*. I'll have a lot to say about both of these points in the opening chapters.

Your teenager may not look exactly like Sara. With almost one teenager in 10 having engaged at least once in what clinicians call "nonsuicidal self-injurious behavior," it's only natural that there would be a wide variation in the behavior and the kids involved with it. Not all teens who self-injure are girls; in fact, there's some evidence that in the general teen population an equal percentage of boys and girls self-injure. In research samples of children who come to clinics, however, girls are much more likely to be in treatment for it. Therefore, I will usually refer to children who self-injure as females. Kids have discovered a variety of ways to self-injure: with razors, scissors, pop-tops from cans, fingernails, bits of glass, and even broken CDs. For some adolescents it is a one- or two-time thing; others will do it many times. As I mentioned, deliberate self-harm often starts in early adolescence, but I have consulted with children who started self-harming as early as 10 years old. Without effective treatment the behavior can persist well into adulthood.

As you will come to see, deliberate self-harm is often a solution to how your child feels in the moment. It can become a stable way of managing painful emotions or a way to escape an awful feeling of numbness and emptiness. Interestingly enough, self-injury does not usually occur in the context of abusing substances, and frequently the adolescent does not feel pain at the moment of injury. Drugs and alcohol often serve a similar function, which might account for why they don't often appear in concert with self-harm.

MARIE: "SOMETIMES I DON'T FEEL ANYTHING AT ALL"

Knowing that you're not alone with this issue probably doesn't make it any less worrisome, frightening, or confusing—especially if you can't find effective treatment, as happened to Marie's mother and father.

"It looks like you're thrilled to be here," I said to Marie in my office.

"I hate shrinks," she replied.

Marie was an attractive young woman with purple hair and several face piercings. She was 17 years old, was date raped at 15, and has a long history of failed psychological treatments. She had had six inpatient admissions at local hospitals for cutting and two for overdosing on pills. She'd gone through seven therapists in the last 4 years. In addition, Marie had spent 9 months in one of the best long-term residential placements in the country. When she left there, she and her parents were quite hopeful about the progress she had made. She had stopped cutting and no longer felt that suicide was an option in her life. The gains she made when living away from home, however, disappeared upon her return. Clearly everybody was disappointed that Marie seemed to be right back where she started.

Her last therapist described her as "unwilling to get better" and as someone who appeared to like the role of patient. He referred her to me, but was clear that he felt she wasn't ready to engage in therapy. It wasn't too hard for me to imagine that Marie could be pretty stubborn. The therapist suggested that she cut to let people see how awful she felt about herself, and that self-injury had the added benefit of helping her receive attention from her friends.

"So why did you come today?" I continued.

With a scowl on her face she grumbled, "They made me."

"And you do everything they tell you?" I asked innocently.

At this point Marie's father interjected that if Marie doesn't start to "get her act together," he was going to send her back to the long-term residential placement where she had done so much better. While clearly he was fed up and at his wit's end, it also seemed that he'd be willing to do whatever it took to help his kid. His statement was not so much a threat as an expression of his ongoing concern, perhaps an indication of how fearful he felt about his daughter's future. Unfortunately, Marie heard it only as a threat and slumped deeper into her chair.

I asked Marie's dad how he understood her problems. Without missing a beat he told me with certainty that her problem is that she keeps trying to get attention. He understood that the date rape may have been a factor in how she felt about herself, but if she just had a little more willpower about putting the past behind her, he said, she wouldn't allow herself to suffer so much. Marie's mother chimed in that her daughter has always been rather "dramatic" and overly sensitive, and while in some ways they are alike in that regard, she has done everything she could for her daughter and is running out of energy. She exclaimed that she has no idea what's going on with her child and burst into tears. Marie expressed her annoyance at having come to this "stupid" appointment and threatened to leave.

I asked Marie if she could stay for just a few more minutes, as I had a couple of questions to ask her. She reluctantly agreed to stay put for the moment.

I was relieved that Marie agreed to stay because there were some important questions that I needed to get answers to right up front. The first was about her experience of cutting and of overdosing. I wanted to determine if cutting and overdosing were similar or different ways of helping her cope. I told her that I was going to ask her a few questions that called for her opinion about herself, then I plunged in.

"When you cut yourself, is your goal to die?"

"No!" she replied without hesitation and with a hint of annoyance.

"I didn't think so," I responded.

"What about when you overdosed? Did you intend to die then?"

"Yes," she mumbled. "I couldn't stand it anymore."

"So for you, cutting serves a different purpose than overdosing. Is that right? Cutting solves the problem of how you feel in the moment, and overdosing is about ending it all."

"Yeah, that's right."

"Okay, Marie, just a few more questions. When you think about yourself compared to others, do you think you are more sensitive than most people?"

"Definitely," she said.

"Do you think it takes longer for you to get over an emotional situation than other people? Do people tend to tell you things like 'Get over it already, you're stewing over something that happened days ago?'" The briefest of smiles and the beginning of some curiosity crossed her face as she responded, "Yes."

"And finally, do you respond really quickly to emotional situations? That is, you know what you feel about something almost immediately, and if you can't name the feeling you still know you feel something very strongly?"

"Totally, but sometimes I don't feel anything at all. I just feel numb and empty," she replied.

I asked her when she feels numb and empty if cutting makes her feel alive again. In other words, does it seem to bring her feelings back?

"Yes!" she replied.

The story about Marie highlights a couple of important points about self-injury in addition to what Sara's story revealed. First, teenagers often have a different intention when they deliberately self-injure than when their intention is suicide. *It is critical that a thorough suicide assessment be conducted by a mental health professional whenever self-injury is part of the picture.* It is equally important that self-injury not get mixed up as suicide because in some important ways each requires a different treatment approach.

The second point is the contention that self-injury is a deliberate attempt by the adolescent to get attention. In my experience this is one of the most frequent misconceptions about self-injury. Parents and therapists alike hold to this misunderstanding as they struggle to understand a very worrisome and perplexing behavior. I discuss both of these points in greater detail in Chapter 1.

WHY DO THEY DO IT?

If it's not a cry for attention, then why do teenagers hurt themselves intentionally? The two most common reasons for self-injuring are (1) to control the extremely painful and frightening experience of overwhelming emotions, and/or (2) to escape from an awful feeling of being numb and empty. Unfortunately, it may not be easy to see that this is what's going on with your son or daughter. A teen who goes straight to her room after school may not reveal the roiling emotion that's tormenting her at the moment. And even if your teen has directly expressed the feeling of emptiness, you may not be able to tell exactly when she's experiencing it. So you're left confounded by the cutting or burning, feeling helpless and profoundly worried.

The paradox of self-injury is that what normally brings pain brings immediate emotional relief in these cases. The key concept in understanding self-injury for the vast majority of teens is that it is an emotional coping strategy. (There are adolescents who self-injure for other reasons, but they form a relatively small group.) Furthermore, as a short-term strategy to manage awful emotional experiences, it can be very effective. It's certainly not an acceptable strategy, but understanding how it serves this function is a critically important first step.

When you—and your teen's therapist—understand that your teen self-injures to get immediate relief from emotional pain or discomfort, you can start solving the problem. But without that understanding therapies may move in the wrong direction, leaving even the most competent therapist, the struggling adolescent, and the most dedicated parent feeling hopeless and frustrated. Professional help you've sought before may have led nowhere, and your own repeated pleas to your teen for an explanation of why she's doing this horrible thing to herself can lead you right down the rabbit hole. My goal in this book is to keep you from falling into it.

Understanding your child's worrisome behavior will help you in two important ways. First, it will lessen your own anxiety. When we understand something, our fear and worry usually decrease. Don't expect to become calm about your kid's trouble, but odds are, once you understand it, you won't panic as much. In addition, it will help you locate appropriate treatment and be better able to assess whether progress is being made.

WHAT YOU CAN DO

Like Sara and Marie, teenagers who self-injure often describe feeling as if they are losing their minds or spinning out of control. To the outside observer it sometimes seems that these kids are being overly dramatic, throwing a tantrum, or making an emotional mountain out of an inconsequential molehill. But being overwhelmed by emotions or not having his or her own emotions available to him or her can have an impact on every aspect of your adolescent's life, from friendships to a sense of identity to what is sometimes described as "impulsive" behavior. Adolescents who cut, or who deliberately self-injure in other ways, lack the skills necessary to manage their feelings. Furthermore, their emotional systems are more highpowered than most people's. They feel things very deeply. Even those who feel numb or empty have usually unconsciously flipped a switch to turn off the very intense feelings that tend to overtake them.

Self-injury is a way to regain emotional balance—it is a solution to the extremely disturbing emotional problem of feeling out of control—*and it works*. It's critical that you understand that fact because it explains why your teen, like Sara, may not really want to stop the cutting. Why? It's like aspirin.

What do you do when you get a headache? You take a pain reliever. What happens? Your headache goes away. How much time do you spend after the relief thinking about why you got a headache? Not much. It seems just human nature that when we solve a problem, we don't spend too much time thinking about why it occurred. The same is true for self-injurers: once the problem (overwhelming emotion or devastating numbness) is solved, they go on with their lives. All too often they don't devote any attention to understanding what set them off and/or developing the skill sets to solve the initial problem.

It is the purpose of this book to explain how your child can develop these skills and how you can reinforce them at home. The first section, "Understanding Self-Injury," lays to rest several popular myths about why adolescents self-injure and introduces you to the facts about this worrisome practice, the factors that lead up to it, and the treatment that works best to help your child overcome it. In the second section, "Helping Your Teen in Treatment and at Home," I go into greater detail about how DBT works and how I conduct this therapy, offering concrete suggestions about what you can do to help your child and to avoid making the situation worse. I'll also give you some pointers about how to remain relatively sane through the tough times. Taking care of yourself is a critical piece of the healing process. Finally, I'll discuss figuring out how, and with whom, to share the problem.

DBT is not a "quick fix." Many adolescents reduce or stop self-injuring in 3 to 6 months, but you will probably need to make a commitment of 1 year. Whether your child stops self-injuring altogether depends on other factors as well, such as his or her support system. As a type of cognitive-behavioral therapy, DBT does not require any special ability or insight. What it requires is recognizing the purpose the behavior has been serving and making a commitment to learning and practicing different ways of soothing a high-powered emotional system. Armed with knowledge and willingness, your child can learn to get past this very difficult time. And you can help. Reading this book is an important start.

PART I

understanding self-injury

I

fact versus fiction

BRINGING SELF-INJURY INTO THE LIGHT

Caitlin's parents were at their wit's end. Whose wouldn't be? Their daughter had been cutting herself several times a week for the past year and a half. All their well-intended attempts at helping her had failed.

"I just don't know what to do at this point," said Caitlin's dad. "We've tried everything: individual therapy, family therapy, all sorts of different medications. We even sent her to a different school. We tried grounding her. We got so desperate we even locked up all the sharp objects in the house. Nothing has worked. I don't think she wants to stop—she must like the attention or something."

Caitlin's mom chimed in: "She's such a good kid. I know she's unhappy. I just wish that she and her therapist could find the reason for her cutting. What does it mean to her? I think if she knew why she did it, she'd be able to stop."

Most of the parents who have sought my consultation, like you, have been caring and loving people who are frustrated and worried sick. It's hard to stay calm when your children seem to be stuck in scary behavior. You experience strong emotions that feel nearly unbearable. And when you're emotionally aroused in this way, the climate is right for you to make errors in thinking and judgment. Your need for answers to aid you through these troubled times can lead you to cling to erroneous conclusions that help lower your anxiety and make sense of the emotional chaos but take you off the right path.

This atmosphere of confusion and misunderstanding has given rise to numerous myths that circulate among lay people and in the media. Therapists themselves have contributed to these myths in some cases because they've been struggling with a problem behavior that has been illuminated by very little scientific research.

Gaining a new understanding of why your children would do something so inconceivable as cutting themselves is much more important than you may believe right now. Of course, you may be much more interested in getting straight to what you can do to make this behavior stop. But acquiring a new perspective on the purpose that self-injury serves for your child is an important foundation for eliminating this disturbing behavior. A new perspective will direct you to effective treatment and help you to facilitate change in your child's behavior by doing some things differently yourself. That's why in this chapter we will examine some of the myths and misconceptions you might have about self-injury and some of the paths you may find yourself going down that keep you from truly understanding the troubles your child is having. The many misunderstandings that parents, pediatricians, and therapists have about deliberate self-harm are a primary reason why children don't get appropriate treatment in a timely way.

Consider Cynthia, a 22-year-old college student who has engaged in self-injurious behavior since the age of 13. Over the weekend Cynthia's roommate noticed the cuts on her arm and told the dorm counselor. Cynthia came to my office only because her dean ordered her to get a psychological consultation before she would be allowed to return to the dormitory.

"I've had therapy since I was a kid, and it hasn't helped with the cutting," Cynthia told me. "I've just become resigned to the fact that this is part of my life. You know, when I cut myself it really doesn't hurt, but it just seems to help. I'm not even sure I want to stop anymore."

"Cutting has been part of your life for almost a decade," I said. "You have been clear with me how it helps you calm down, so I can imagine you have mixed feelings about giving it up."

"Yes, in some ways it's like an old friend who is a bit troublesome but who is always there when you need her."

Cynthia's a little older than the patients I usually see. For the most part in this book I will be talking about teenagers, because the vast majority of people who engage in deliberate self-harm begin it in adolescence—and that's when you're most likely to be trying to understand and eliminate it from your child's life. I want to leave no doubt in your mind that you should seek professional help for your child if you know, or reading this book confirms your suspicion, that your teenager has been engaging in self-injury. While some kids only experiment with the behavior, for most it will continue into the early adult years and even into midlife and beyond unless prompt and effective psychological treatment is sought. That can be difficult to pursue when misconceptions get in the way.

MYTHS ABOUT SELF-INJURY

Please keep the following ideas in mind when you read about these myths. First, in psychology nothing is absolute or certain, so in a few instances what is a *myth* when applied to an entire population can be a *fact* in an individual case. Second, most of our behavior is influenced by many factors, including our past history, our current needs, and our long- and short-term goals. Not all these factors have an equal influence. Some have a minor role in keeping the behavior going, while others exert a powerful effect.

Myth 1: They Do It to Get Attention

According to some researchers, less than 4% of adolescents deliberately hurt themselves to get attention. Yet it's the most common reason that parents and some therapists give to account for the behavior—despite the fact that often an adolescent is self-injuring for months before an adult even notices. Misconceptions of this kind derail treatment and prolong both the adolescent's and the parents' distress, as it did for Erin and her family.

ERIN: NOT FOR ATTENTION

Erin, age 13, was a very likable and extremely bright girl who seemed to have some anxiety in social situations. She had been hospitalized numerous times over the last 6 months for self-injury and suicidal thinking. The psychiatrist in charge of her care reported that Erin had been cutting herself for the past 2 years, but that it had come to her parents' attention only about 8 months ago. When I asked the psychiatrist if he had any ideas about why Erin injured herself, he replied with confidence that he, the previous clinicians, and Erin's parents were all convinced that she did it to get attention.

How could a young girl be seeking attention through a behavior that she kept secret for well over a year? When I posed this question to the psychiatrist, he realized immediately that he may have leapt too quickly to his conclusion. So how is it that smart, well-trained, competent clinicians and caring, loving parents so often make this mistake? It's hard to know for sure, but here are some possibilities.

Even "Delicate Cutting" Is Self-Soothing

First, the majority of self-injurious behavior involves relatively superficial wounds. Some clinicians refer to superficial cutting or scratching as "delicate cutting"—giving the impression that the adolescent is taking care not to hurt herself seriously, but only to cause enough damage to get people to notice. But these superficial wounds have the self-soothing effect that these adolescents seek. (I discuss the smaller group of more serious self-injurers later in this chapter.)

Parents' Proximity

A second reason why parents might get off track about self-injury has to do with the context in which the behavior occurs. Once you realize that your child is self-injuring, you will probably become more vigilant about her mood changes and emotional states, thus keeping you near your child. If she hurts herself when you're close, it would be easy to assume she did it to capture your attention. Many parents have told me how they know their child is having emotional trouble, but when they try to help, the child often rebukes them or denies that anything is wrong. The parents know that this is untrue and so they stay close at hand. In a matter of minutes the child self-injures right in the next room, and the parents rush in to help. The child is a little calmer now and somewhat more willing to talk. The parents conclude that she hurt herself to get the attention she is now willing to accept.

Parents are often both relieved and annoyed by this sequence of events—relieved that their child was open with them but annoyed because they felt manipulated by the behavior. They conclude that the self-injury is a manipulative ploy to get them to pay attention. Their frustration is compounded because of their thwarted attempts to help.

There's another explanation for this sequence of events.

Adolescents Want Privacy

The alternative explanation rests on two factors. The first is the normal tendency for adolescents to seek privacy concerning their emotional lives. This is especially true for those in the early to middle stages of adolescence. For boys, early to midadolescence ranges from 13 to 16 years of age; for girls it's a little earlier, from 11 to 15. Hallmarks of this stage of development are the phrases "I don't want to talk about it" and "Everything is fine"—the second of which often doesn't square with what you see.

At this point in their lives, adolescents feel a real need to be separate and independent from their parents. As they negotiate these new waters, they often confuse asking for help with child-like dependency. These kids pull hard against any current that might make them feel like a younger child. They have not learned to differentiate between mature dependency, which includes the capacity to ask for help and advice, and a pseudoindependence that places a premium on going it alone. For the most part, kids in this stage of development try to keep their parents out of their business. While they may wear outlandish clothes and behave in ways that are "over the top," they rarely intend to promote tighter scrutiny from their parents. Ironically, it is just such behavior that often invites adults in to set limits.

> *At an age when their mantras are "I don't want to talk about it" and "Everything's fine," teenagers rarely seek parental attention—much less help.*

More Emotion Than They Can Handle

The second point that supports an alternative explanation for Erin's behavior has to do with the way these kids experience emotional distress. By and large, adolescents who self-injure are extremely reactive people: they feel things very deeply and are prone to becoming emotionally overwhelmed quickly. They possess powerful emotional systems without the tools to manage them—it's as if they have Ferrari engines and Toyota Corolla transmissions. They have great difficulty harnessing their powerful emotions in the service of clear thinking and problem solving. When they're emotionally charged up, they lack the capacity to skillfully ask for help or to take in new information that may alleviate their current distress. What they want to solve, and to solve quickly, is how awful they feel in the moment.

> *Kids who self-injure have the emotional engine of a Ferrari with the transmission of a Toyota Corolla.*

Self-injury often provides immediate relief from this feeling of emotional turmoil. With that relief comes a degree of calmness that enables them to be more available and reasonable with their parents. The change in demeanor, coupled with the parents' presence, makes it seem as if they injured themselves to get attention, but it's almost always about getting immediate relief from emotional distress. (Those cases where it doesn't provide emotional relief are discussed in Chapter 3.)

Myth 2: Everyone's Doing It

Deliberate self-injury has been part of the adolescent scene for many years. My clinical experience and that of my colleagues suggest that it's on the rise, but we don't know for sure. We are uncertain for at least three reasons.

Deliberate Self-Injury Has Often Been Mistakenly Documented as a Suicide Attempt

Since suicide attempts appear to be on the rise, when self-injury gets mistaken for attempted suicide, it seems erroneously that self-injury is on the rise. Marie's story from the Introduction highlights the different experience teens have when they are actively suicidal, as opposed to using self-injury to soothe themselves.

I can't emphasize enough the importance of a thorough assessment by a qualified mental health professional to sort out this issue. Most of the adolescents I treat are quite clear about how different these two experiences feel for them. (Often the adults around them, who are worried, baffled, and at their wit's end, are inadvertently generating the confusion.) They tell me that they deliberately self-injure when they just can't stand how painful life feels a minute longer. They may wish they were dead, but they have no intention of killing themselves. In contrast, when they are feeling suicidal, they do intend to end their lives. But don't try to make this distinction in your own children. Seek a professional's help.

No Firm Criteria

Some researchers employ a rather narrow view of what constitutes nonsuicidal self-injury while others use the broadest of criteria. Consequently, the percentages given for adolescents in the general population who self-injure range from 9 to 39%; for adolescents who are hospitalized for psychiatric reasons, the range is 40 to 61%. As clinicians' and researchers' attention is drawn more and more to this area, I believe it won't be too long before we have more definitive answers to these questions.

Today's Kids Seem Less Secretive about It

While we don't know for sure whether self-injury is on the rise, in my experience adolescents used to be more secretive about it in years past; it would have been unusual for a child to speak about such behavior even to his closest friend. Parents often remained unaware of a child's self-injury until his psychiatric hospitalization for some other reason. As time went on, stories of self-injury crept into the media, both in news reports about teenage health issues and in the adolescent music and movie culture. In a way self-injury has been "normalized." As a consequence, adolescents are much more likely to disclose their self-injurious behavior to friends and to discuss how it makes them feel better in the short run. In addition, a number of Internet sites are devoted to self-injury. We don't know whether these sites help children to stop self-injury or induce them to keep it up, but it's another route by which self-injury has "come out of the closet."

The good news with self-injury coming out of the closet is that researchers began to study the problem in an attempt both to understand it and to develop more effective treatments. The not-so-good news is that as more adolescents became aware of the behavior, more tried it out in a moment of emotional turmoil. Unfortunately, for a significant number of adolescents, the behavior worked all too well in helping them regain their psychological equilibrium. In the media and in the adolescent culture, self-injury is often portrayed in ways that glamorize or romanticize it rather than address its devastating long-term consequences. You may even have come to believe from these portrayals that self-injury is a worrisome behavior that your children will outgrow once they're out of their teens. Sadly, this is not true. The child who self-injures is in significant emotional distress and needs professional guidance.

Myth 3: Peer Pressure Is the Main Culprit

While kids who cut themselves are often friends with other adolescents who do the same, peer pressure probably has little effect on keeping the behavior going. For adolescents, and in particular female teenagers, the peer group is a place to air their problems. It's not unusual for one teenager to tell another about her personal experience with self-injury or to let on that another friend has tried it. Teens can also find out about it from the media. In fact, preliminary data suggest that about 52% of kids learn about self-injury from a friend or the media.

Peer Pressure as Scapegoat

Peer pressure has been used to explain many kinds of adolescent behavior, often without merit. For example, it's often been cited as a reason adolescents use alcohol and drugs. While peer pressure can probably make someone use these substances on a few occasions, it's more typical for kids who are involved in substance use or abuse to seek each other out, thereby creating a new peer group. A similar pattern probably occurs with self-injury.

As adolescents describe it, only their friends have the insight and ability to understand and help them. It's true that cliques are an important part of adolescent life, and I don't want to downplay the importance of a child's feeling of belonging and support. I find, however, that a social group offers its members an abundance of understanding and compassion but not much in the way of helping one another change undesirable behaviors. The problem is more likely to be solved from the inside out: when kids stop self-injuring, they will be more likely to find new friends, rather than new friends in their group somehow helping them to stop self-injuring, as Melanie's story shows.

MELANIE: "I LIKE THESE NEW FRIENDS BETTER"

Melanie had been in treatment for 8 months and hadn't cut herself for the past three. She started the session with an upbeat story about a concert she had attended with some friends.

"Did you go with Dee and Nick?" I asked.

"No, I actually don't see them much anymore," she replied.

"I know your parents worked very hard to stop you from hanging out with them. Is that why?"

"No way," she told me. "When they wouldn't let me see them, I just did it behind their backs. I don't pick their friends, why should they pick mine? They thought I was being influ-

> *Adolescents generally don't start injuring themselves because of the influence of friends. They are more likely to choose friends who share their behavior.*

enced by Dee and Nick, like I don't have a brain of my own. I don't know, I just feel like I'm changing and I like these new friends better."

Myth 4: Drugs and Alcohol Increase the Likelihood of Self-Injury

Self-injury soothes emotional distress, just as drugs and alcohol do. So the behavior, especially in a child who self-injures as a way to regulate emotions, would rarely be triggered by drug or alcohol use. What happened to Vicki illustrates how they serve the same purpose.

I had been meeting in dialectical behavioral therapy for the last 4 months with Vicki, a 16-year-old high school junior. She came to therapy for cutting, but she often also had problems with drinking. As we worked on reducing her self-injury, we noticed that she began drinking more.

"You know, I think I might be drinking as a substitute for cutting," she told me in one session.

"I think you're on to something, since both behaviors seem to be geared toward helping you feel less anxious around friends," I replied. "I think we better target your drinking along with your cutting behavior."

The exception is the relatively small group of self-injurers who hurt themselves from severe self-hatred and contempt and for whom self-injury is about relieving guilt through physical pain. These children have often suffered sexual abuse, and they're more likely to harm themselves in the context of substance use.

John, a 19-year-old college freshman, came in to talk with me about his self-injurious behavior. He had been sexually abused by a cousin from age 7 to age 11. John prided himself on his academics and had done very well through High School.

"I never cut myself before. It just seemed to start around exam time first semester. I put a lot of pressure on myself to perform, and I was really stressed out," he told me.

"Tell me about the first time," I prodded.

"I was studying for my math final. I'm usually very good at math, but I just couldn't seem to get the concepts. One night I just got really frustrated and began to drink in my room. The next thing I knew, I just was feeling all this intense self–hatred. Without thinking I picked up my X-Acto knife and began cutting."

Myth 5: Certain Kids Manage Physical Pain More Easily Than Emotional Pain

Frequently when I ask adolescents about their self-injurious behavior, they tell me that it's easier for them to bear physical pain than emotional pain. Like an alchemist of old, they claim to be able to turn emotional pain into physical pain. It does seem like a good idea to change a problem you can't solve into one that you can. But when I ask them if their self-injurious behavior hurts, typically the answer is no. So how can it be easier to manage physical pain than emotional pain if there is no physical pain? I'm convinced from my numerous discussions with these kids that they are not deliberately distorting their experience. How can we reconcile this seeming conundrum?

When emotionally revved up, some people experience a sense of calmness and relief when they damage their skin tissue.

In all likelihood the mechanism that provides the relief for these children has to do with the neuropsychological effect of self-injury some people experience when they are in an intense emotional state. This sense of soothing is the most common experience that kids have at the moment of self-injury. While we do not yet have a full understanding of how this works, it seems that some people, when emotionally revved up, experience a sense of calmness and relief when they damage skin tissue. This may have to do with a kind of opiate-like endorphin that is released at the moment of tissue damage. These kids, however, explain their experience in a different way: they claim that physical pain is easier to manage than emotional pain.

The Mustard Test

Psychologists and marketing professionals both know that the reasons people give for their behavior and the true motivation behind it are often two very different kettles of fish. If you place a particular brand of mustard on the top corner shelf in a grocery store, for example, and then ask people why they bought that brand, they may tell you it's because of its fabulous taste. If you then put that brand on the bottom shelf, the very same customers might buy a different brand now sitting on the top corner shelf. If you ask them why they bought the second brand, they may tell you it's because of its wonderful taste. Clearly, though, the mustard's place on the shelf was what determined which brand customers purchased.

Psychologists have developed something called "attribution theory" as a way to explain this kind of behavior. Simply put, *attribution theory* examines the ways in which our beliefs are related or unrelated to why we do the things we do, and how our beliefs can influence our behavior and our sense of ourselves. Our attributions can be divided into two categories. *Internal attributions* comprise our beliefs about what kind of person we are, and *external attributions* focus on our beliefs about factors that influence our behavior from the outside. For example, if I run in a race and I do well, I may tell myself that I did well because I trained hard and that I am naturally gifted. This would be an example of an internal attribution. On the other hand, if I tell myself that I did well because the field of runners that day was poor, that would be an example of an external attribution. So how might all this relate to our dilemma?

When adolescents tell me they experience no pain at the time of self-injury but that they self-injure because they manage physical pain better than emotional pain, I gently point out the contradiction to help them begin to see that other factors may be at work. These kids believe (and it's true) that they can't effectively manage emotional pain, which they often experience as a personal weakness. Believing that they can manage physical pain is a positive aspect of their personality, and so they trick themselves into believing that their self-injury is a strategy to harness a positive aspect of their personality. They explain their behavior based on the internal attribution that they can manage physical pain more competently than emotional pain. While this explanation has some validity, it doesn't accurately or fully explain their self-injury.

Myth 6: It's a Failed Suicide Attempt

If I had written this book 10 or 15 years ago, Myth 6 would have been first on the list. Thankfully, most clinicians now are better able to differentiate self-injury from self-harm with the intent to die. This determination can be a complex clinical endeavor, however, and the bottom line is that if you're worried, you should get your child evaluated. Most kids who are suicidal let someone close to them know about it. The notion that if someone were really going to kill himself he wouldn't tell anyone is a myth. Furthermore, as you well know, things can change pretty rapidly with teenagers, so even if you had a consultation, get another one if your worry comes back.

Suicide is the third leading cause of death among adolescents (after car accidents and murder). While we have some clear ideas about risk factors for suicide, many kids have risk factors and never make a suicide attempt. What is terribly clear, however, is that the single most powerful risk factor that predicts future suicidal behavior is a past attempt. See the accompanying box of other risk factors. See also the list in Chapter 3 of self-injuring behaviors that may predispose an adolescent to suicide attempts.

More often than not, deliberate self-harm is not a failed or half-hearted suicide attempt. But as with Marie, described in the Introduction, some kids have both experienced suicidal thoughts *and* injured themselves. And then there are kids who injure themselves as a type of suicide prevention. As I mentioned before, only a qualified mental health professional can make this determination. It's critical that any child who is self-injuring undergo a thorough suicide assessment by a qualified professional. If your child is struggling with suicide, your treatment team and you will need to stay vigilant about any evidence of worsening mood, talk of hopelessness, or references to wanting to die.

RISK FACTORS FOR SUICIDE

1. Psychological troubles like major depression, bipolar disorder, borderline personality disorder, or anxiety disorders.
2. Substance use.
3. Severe family problems.
4. A recent loss—for example, a break-up of a romantic relationship, a move, or a change in school.
5. The recent suicide of another adolescent in the community.
6. Impulsive or risky behaviors.
7. Self-injury.
8. Struggling with issues about sexual orientation.

A NEW APPROACH TO UNDERSTANDING WHY YOUR CHILD IS SELF-INJURING

For children to hurt themselves in an attempt to feel better is so counterintuitive that it's only natural to look for an explanation beneath the surface. Surely something else—some hidden, unresolved need—must be causing the behavior. But the search for such hidden meaning has given rise to many of the myths just discussed. It has also led therapists away from a key concept: hurting themselves does make some kids feel better in a very specific way at the moment they do it.

Since the time of Sigmund Freud, psychologists have been interested in the *meaning* hidden in a person's actions. This kind of detective work can be an important tool in psychotherapy, but it can lead therapists and patients on a wild goose chase where self-injury is concerned. Recognizing the *function* of these kids' self-harm, rather than trying to ferret out a symbolic *meaning*, is the new understanding that makes it possible to help them give up this behavior. When we understand the purpose their self-harm has been serving, we can help kids find a healthier way to serve the same purpose—both in treatment and in support of that treatment at home.

Let me give you an example.

TAMAR AND THE PUPPY

Tamar is a very bright college student who has a long history of self-injury and eating-disordered behavior. She has had several tries at more conventional individual talk therapies aimed at helping her understand the meaning of her eating-disordered behavior. Her parents divorced when she was in elementary school. Her mother and father are two high-powered professionals who travel often as part of their work. While Tamar had a good relationship with her parents, she felt they pressured her to conform to their ideas of success. Her eating-disordered behavior reached a level where she couldn't remain at college and had to return to live with her mother, although she often spent time at her father's house. After several hospitalizations, she began outpatient psychotherapy with me. An especially difficult problem for Tamar was binge eating in the middle of the night. At one point she had made some gains in this area by using skills she had learned in therapy with me, but we were not sure what *triggered* the behavior or what *function* it served for her. About 3 months into our meetings, she began to backslide. It was a puzzle to both of us.

She started one of her sessions by saying, "I think I know why I started to binge again. It has to do with my father coming home from his business trips.

I get really tense when he's home. I just know that he wishes I would get my act together. He doesn't understand how much I'm struggling."

As the therapy hour progressed, I learned that Tamar had recently acquired a puppy that she was in the process of housebreaking. As part of the training, Tamar would get up in the middle of the night to take the puppy outside. She told me that she was always fearful of waking her father on these late-night trips with the puppy. Furthermore, she complained of how intolerant her parents were of her puppy's behavior and said she would become stressed and tense in response to their criticisms. What we learned when we went step by step looking at what happened when she took the puppy out was the following.

Tamar would get extremely tense when she noticed that her puppy might have to go out. As we talked, she realized that when she went down the stairs and out the front door she didn't binge, but when she went down the stairs and out the back door through the kitchen, she did. It seemed that seeing the refrigerator was the trigger for bingeing. If she didn't see the refrigerator, she stood a better chance of accessing her new skills to help her manage her stress. The function of her bingeing, it became clear, was to reduce her stress. The remedy, then, was simply to go out the front door.

This is the same type of solution that becomes accessible in treating self-injury when we look at its function rather than try to discover its buried meaning. With the trigger out of the picture and a better understanding of the function her bingeing had for her, we were able to develop a treatment strategy that would make Tamar's bingeing a thing of the past. If I had focused exclusively on the *meaning* of Tamar's bingeing in relation to the complicated feelings she had about her father, her eating disorder would no doubt have continued much longer. I had to assess the *function* of Tamar's behavior and also work at understanding her beliefs about the behavior.

When speaking with your child's therapist, listen carefully to how the clinician is thinking about your child's self-injury so that you can differentiate the meaning of a behavior from its function. The accompanying box will help you accomplish this.

---

1. To find the *meaning* of the behavior, ask "Why?" Answers are generally: "I cut myself because I hate myself," or "I deserve to be punished," or "She needs to show people how much she hurts."
2. To find the *function* of the behavior, ask "What reinforces the behavior?" The most frequent answer to that question is that it changes the individual's painful emotional state, providing some sense of relief.

The Road to a New Therapy

The psychological theories that informed most of my earlier career were variations on psychoanalytic concepts first proposed by Freud, then refined and expanded over the years by many of his followers. As I mentioned, this kind of therapy is very useful for some kinds of psychological problems, but did not prove useful for the adolescents I was seeing who were self-harming. My task as a therapist at that time was to help my patients understand the reasons and meaning behind their behavior. I saw a person's troubled behavior as a symptom of some deeper underlying psychological problem. The idea here was that if I could help my patients understand the meaning of their behavior, or develop insight, it would lead them to confront that underlying issue. They would then be better able to choose a more adaptive way of managing and resolving what was troubling them.

The problem was that unearthing buried psychological problems so that the teenager could develop insight took a very long time—time during which the teen's self-destructive behavior continued. To make matters worse, it wasn't always possible to find the right insight or combination of insights that would aid the child in recovery. The adolescent and the therapist might examine the recurrent patterns in the child's relationships with friends, for example. The goal would be for the adolescent to understand what specific needs are not being met in these relationships and how the child is contributing to this problem. The idea is that with this insight, the child can alter his or her friendship patterns, thus reducing negative emotions that lead to self-harm. A more direct approach would involve the therapist and the teen monitoring and addressing the child's self-harming behavior as the problem that must be solved first.

Good therapists, however, have been taking the more indirect route for years with reasonable results. My own experience is that the more indirect tactics, while viable, take longer to resolve self-harm behavior. In addition, even when some of the kids had that "Aha!" moment, they didn't have the emotional skills to overcome their problem. I needed a way to help these kids stop hurting themselves as quickly as possible.

When I began to read about a treatment called dialectical behavior therapy, or DBT, I knew it could be the answer I'd been hoping for. DBT has two major strengths (as well as many others, which you'll read about in later chapters) that address self-injury effectively and efficiently:

1. *It targets the problematic behavior directly.* It does not spend time seeking out hidden meanings or ask the teen or anyone else to attribute the behavior to symbolic motivations. It looks directly at what self-injury does for

the teen when she does it and gives her other ways to serve the same purpose. As I'll explain further in Chapter 2 and beyond, the purpose self-injury serves is the obvious one, as counterintuitive as it may seem: At the moment when your teenager does it, cutting or burning herself makes her feel better, not physically but *emotionally*.

2. *DBT recognizes that conflict between the teen, who finds self-injury useful, and the parents and therapist, who want the behavior to stop, erects a major obstacle to change*. Misconceptions and conflicting viewpoints about self-injury generate tense and ineffective relationships in therapy. You're undoubtedly well aware that they cause unnecessary distress between you and your child. The "dialectic" in DBT is a way of finding a middle ground where you (and the therapist) can work toward change. On the one hand, you convey to the teen that you understand her emotional pain and her need to relieve it, while on the other hand, you nudge her toward eliminating self-injury by giving her new ways to alleviate the pain.

I hope you can see from this simplified explanation that DBT is nothing if not practical. The goal for DBT therapists is the same as it is for you: to help your teenager stop hurting herself. The element that you've been lacking so far is the "how." DBT supplies that by offering your teen better ways to ease her emotional pain. This book will show you how you can adopt DBT's principles and strategies to contribute to such efforts made in treatment. But first, let me introduce a couple of teenagers who illustrate the two points just introduced.

AISHA: WEAVING TOGETHER MULTIPLE POINTS OF VIEW

It's difficult to bear the uncertainty about what guides the troubled actions of our loved ones. In these moments we're likely to jump to conclusions. Our thinking tends to become rigid and constricted, so we can't take in additional information that could help us. We can also lose our ability to logically sort things out, so we become overwhelmed and helpless. As much as we want to do something, anything, to help our suffering child, inertia more often than not wins out.

To complicate things even more, you and your child's other parent may not be on the same page. Often one parent's thinking becomes rigid and constricted while the other parent feels emotionally overwhelmed, which can lead to an ineffective parenting approach: "Houston, we have a problem." The single parent faces much the same dilemma, alternating between hopelessness and a rigid certainty in thinking—neither of which can help the suffering child. My work with Aisha is a good example of how things can get derailed and how to get them back on track.

Fifteen-year-old Aisha lived with her dad, stepmother, and younger brother and sister. She had minimal contact with her mother, who lived in another state. Aisha's stepmom had worked hard to forge a relationship with her, and in many ways has been successful in negotiating these very tricky waters. As every stepparent knows, this is not an easy task. After the stepmom had been in the house for a while and things seemed to be settling down, she decided to pursue an advanced degree in business. This had been a dream of hers for several years, which she had put on hold while she took on the responsibilities of a stepmother. Aisha's stepmother was a confident, nononsense kind of person and she reveled in the demands of graduate school.

Aisha's dad, a quiet and thoughtful man, valued peace and harmony in his family life. He told me that often he was puzzled by his daughter's periodic emotional outbursts, and downright angry about her cutting. I saw Aisha with her father and stepmother in a one-time consultation. Aisha had just returned home after a 5-day inpatient stay that was precipitated by her cutting herself after a family quarrel.

"So does anyone have a theory about what this self-injurious behavior is all about?" I asked.

Almost simultaneously father and stepmother began speaking.

"It's not rocket science, Dr. Hollander," Aisha's father said with a clear tone of frustration and annoyance in his voice. "Aisha picks those times when her stepmom is overloaded with schoolwork and just can't devote the time she usually spends with the kids. It's not easy juggling full-time family obligations with graduate school. She's only human; she can't do everything. Aisha needs to understand that and stop trying to be the center of attention."

Aisha's stepmom went on to say, "It's almost like clockwork. Exam time comes around or I have a paper due, and that's when we can almost count on Aisha finding a way to cut. She is so predictable. She just has to have my attention all the time."

"That's not true!" Aisha sobbed. "I don't want your attention. Stop saying that. I hate the attention I get when I cut. I have tried everything to stop cutting and I just can't do it!"

Clearly Aisha felt misunderstood by her parents, but couldn't offer an alternative explanation for her self-injury. In the absence of another explanation, the parents held tightly to their point of view, leaving Aisha with what appeared to be empty denials. The standoff left everyone feeling frustrated and tense. The more Aisha denied her cutting as a bid for attention, the more her parents leveled evidence to support their point of view.

There had to be more to the story. The parents' theory made good sense, yet Aisha's side was equally compelling. What too often occurs in these conversational standoffs is that each person starts to bring more and more energy and insistence—and loudness—to bolster his or her own position, while the capacity to understand the other person's point of view goes out the window. I imagine that a few of you reading this know all too well what I am describing here.

The key to success in moments like these is for you to stand back and work at gathering more information. I will focus on how to negotiate these tricky moments in later chapters. For now, the essential idea is to become unattached from your point of view and to bring some genuine curiosity and interest to the situation at hand. Give up on being "right." Try instead to develop an effective collaboration on the issues facing you and your child. Work at truly taking in your child's point of view and finding the truth in his or her position. I refer to this as "weaving in multiple points of view." In doing so we are discovering the kernel of truth in each person's perspective and working at bringing it all together to form a more complete view of the situation. You can always come back to your point of view later.

Of course this is easier said than done, especially when your emotions are running high and your children's welfare is at stake. When you can let

> *To form the most complete view of your teen's self-injury, find the kernel of truth in each person's point of view and then bring all of these kernels together.*

go of your piece of the truth and work at developing a more complete view of things, however, I promise you that the tension and frustration will begin to decrease. I've seen it happen again and again. It works best when everybody involved is willing to do the same; but even if just one party makes the shift, it can be beneficial for everybody.

"It seems like you guys are stuck," I said to Aisha's family. "No two ways about it, things can get pretty hectic at home with everybody so busy. What is it like for each of you?"

Aisha's stepmom spoke first: "I do what I can for my family—they really are my first priority—but when my schoolwork requires my attention, it becomes a real tug of war about how I'm going to divide my time. I have to admit, I can get pretty irritable and short on patience in those moments."

Aisha's dad chimed in: "I guess we all start walking on eggshells so as not to disturb my wife during the high-stress periods. You know, one wrong move and she's liable to bite your head off!" he added, only half-joking.

Aisha jumped in: "I really get feeling pretty crazy with all the tension

The key to taking in other points of view to help solve a serious problem is understanding that

1. You may have developed a rigid adherence to your own position.
2. You are not betraying yourself by being curious about other people's opinions.
3. It's of little importance to be "right"; the only thing that matters is gathering information to help solve the crisis.
4. Taking pieces of other people's viewpoints plus pieces of your own, at least temporarily, may yield a fuller picture than any single person's viewpoint can.

when my stepmom is under all that pressure. It seems like the whole house and me included are vibrating with stress. Sometimes I just can't take it."

"Does your cutting give you some relief from all that stress?" I asked.

"Yes!" Aisha answered immediately.

Clearly, it was Aisha's response to the tension in the house rather than her wish for attention that generated her self-injury. Her parents' theory, while in many ways logical, was wrong. In part, their own frustration helped lock them into a logical but false conclusion. Like the majority of adolescents who self-injure, Aisha used cutting as a way to bring relief from the awful emotional tension that she felt inside. Only when her parents were able to re-evaluate their position could they respond to her with genuine empathy. And when they understood the function of her cutting, they could begin to come up with better ways to manage the tension in their household.

JANINE: VALIDATING THE TEEN'S EMOTIONAL EXPERIENCE

As mentioned above, the other major strength of DBT is that it tackles the behavior directly because it is based on understanding that the behavior serves the teen's need to alleviate emotional pain and by giving the teen better ways to meet that need than harming him or herself. The first and most important step toward accomplishing that goal is to ensure that you validate the way your child feels. Janine's story illustrates.

"You just don't get it! Lizzie is my best friend, and she understands me better than anybody else," Janine exclaimed through her tears.

"She's no best friend as far as I'm concerned," countered Janine's dad. "I don't think she's a friend at all! What kind of friend supports you cutting yourself?"

"She doesn't support my cutting. She just talks with me about my problems," Janine explained through her sobs.

This is the beginning of a conversation that is guaranteed to go nowhere. I hope you can recognize the truths in Janine's position and the truths in her father's as well. What is missing in the dialogue is *validation*—that is, communicating that you understand and value the wisdom in the other person's point of view. Validation means communicating that you understand the other person's experience. This doesn't mean that you have to *share* the opinion.

For example, Janine's dad need only say that he understands how valuable Lizzie's friendship is to her.

> *Validation is like fertilizer for relationships—it keeps them growing. It nurtures and enhances the relationship so the more arid times are easier to bear.*

Validation is like fertilizer for relationships: it keeps them growing. It nurtures and enhances them, so the more arid times are easier to bear. Furthermore, after he validates Janine's experience, he will be in a better position to raise his concerns about Lizzie and have them heard. The concept of validation may seem simple, but I have found it to be the single most difficult skill to teach to parents and the most important one for them to acquire.

These brief stories give you a glimpse into why self-injury can be so difficult to eliminate. By its paradoxical nature it creates conflicts and misunderstandings—between parent and child, between parents, and between child and therapist—that can stand in the way of change. You need a way to bridge the gap between opposing points of view if you are to work together toward change. And unless everyone—your teen, you, and the teen's therapist—understands and validates the teen's emotional experience, the teen is not likely to be receptive. If you can't see that she's in a lot of pain and that self-injury is her attempt to soothe herself, why would she trust your advice on how to "get better"? It would be like telling her to throw away her crutches and cut off her cast because you didn't understand that she had broken her leg.

Of course emotional pain isn't visible. Let's move on to a discussion that will bring to light how your child became vulnerable to the emotional pain that urged her to start injuring herself.

2

what sets the stage
for self-injury?

Spend a minute or two thinking about how you would answer these questions:

1. Do you think your child is more sensitive than most?
2. Do you think your child has an immediate and often intense emotional reaction to life events?
3. Does it seem that it takes your child longer than most to get over emotional reactions?
4. Can your teen get all her tasks done when she's in a good mood, but accomplish very little when she's in a bad mood?

My guess is that you would answer "yes" to all these questions, thus describing a person who is emotionally vulnerable and tends to act based on mood. Your child may be self-injuring as a way to regain some emotional balance. In fact, some researchers estimate that's what 80% of kids who self-injure are doing.

But, like many parents, you may notice that your child doesn't seem to feel any emotions at all. "I just can't read her anymore," Ellery's mom told me with concern. "I know she's really upset, but she just doesn't show any emotion. When I ask her how she feels, she just answers 'Fine,' but I know she's hurting."

Some of these children have a sense of dread about directly experiencing their feelings and have developed strategies to avoid them. They're out of touch with their feelings, unable to apply accurate labels to their emotions. They're worried that if they were to feel, they would become emotionally overwhelmed—and they may be right. When asked how they feel, they often quickly answer, "I don't know"—an automatic response that helps them short-circuit any awareness of their emotions.

Others have developed the ability to "mask" their feelings. They usually have some idea about what they're feeling, but for a variety of reasons they don't let on through their facial expressions or words. Avoiding or masking feelings is a strategy that will not work for long. Eventually the emotional tension in these kids becomes unbearable, and that's when they're prone to self-injury.

The recipe for emotional vulnerability calls for two ingredients: emotional reactivity and an environment that has somehow made the kids doubt the validity of their own emotional experiences. When I talk about *emotional reactivity*, I am thinking about three things: first, emotionally reactive people feel things more deeply than most; second, their reaction to emotional stimuli is almost immediate; and third, once they are emotionally aroused, it takes them a longer time than other people to recover. They are often described as "oversensitive," "overly emotional," "high-strung," "temperamental," or even dismissively as "drama queens."

An *environment* that fails to help the child learn how to identify, accurately label, and modulate emotions can arise from a combination of factors in the child's surroundings. Let me make clear that this is rarely the result of inadequate parenting. Rather, the parental strategies of reassurance and problem solving that work in most cases often backfire with these children. You know this only too well: these children are difficult to parent.

> *The typical parental techniques of reassurance and problem solving often fail with emotionally vulnerable kids.*

For example, your daughter may ask you how she looks in her new dress and you tell her honestly that the color is beautiful, but you wonder whether it might be too dressy for the party she's going to. This comment may send her tearfully sulking to her room and refusing to go out, leaving you feeling perplexed, angry, and unfairly blamed.

In this chapter I'll help you learn more about the qualities of emotional reactivity so you can determine whether they are operating in your teenager, as well as about the environmental factors that lead to emotional vulnerabilities. Understanding what happens when these two factors come together puts you in a better position to help your teenager stop self-injuring.

BIOLOGICAL VULNERABILITIES: THE SENSITIVE CHILD

If we were to measure emotional reactivity on a scale, we would most likely find that the majority of people fall in the middle. At one end would be people who are only mildly reactive and on the other end would be the most reactive people. With very few exceptions, one's degree of emotional reactivity is determined by biological makeup, like eye color or natural athletic ability, not by one's environment.

Being emotionally reactive is not necessarily a psychological problem. We all know people who are very sensitive and have learned how to manage their high-powered emotional systems. They tend to be very empathic, to be the kind of friends you would be likely to let in on a personal difficulty. Emotionally reactive people live more in the emotional side of life. But what about those children who haven't acquired the skills to manage their high-powered emotional systems? These are the ones who become emotionally vulnerable. They have a truly hard time tolerating negative emotions like sadness and anger, and they have a hard time finding ways to increase positive emotions like happiness or interest. Researchers have coined the term "emotional dysregulation" to describe how emotionally vulnerable people respond to the experience of negative and positive emotions.

Emotional Dysregulation

"Roberta wasn't always this way," Mrs. Martin explained. "As a child she would certainly have her moments, but since the beginning of adolescence she's a changed person. The slightest thing seems to send her into an emotional tizzy." Roberta's father added: "It's like everything has to be this big drama production, and whatever suggestions you make, she shoots them right down. I know Roberta is unhappy, but you would think she has it worse than anybody. She has no perspective."

People who are not emotionally vulnerable often just can't understand those who are (and vice versa). Not only is it hard to understand why they seem to "overreact" all the time, but their emotional dysregulation can be manifested in so many ways that it's not obvious that it's the central problem behind most self-injurious behavior. For example, the night before midterm exams your son comes home from school and begins to play video games. You have a sense that something's troubling him, but when you question him on his way to his room, he tells you everything is "fine." After the second hour you go into his room and try to talk to him, at which point he tells you that he can't study and he's going to fail anyway. You suggest that if he does study, then maybe he won't fail. He says once again that you don't understand him and tells you to get out of his room. Naturally the situation deteriorates from here with you trying to stay reasonable while he becomes more and more emotionally distraught.

What's really happening here? Your son can't articulate how worried and overwhelmed he feels about his schoolwork and the fact that all his friends seem to be doing better than he is. His worry and his sense of being a poorer student than his friends has put him in a dark mood that cripples him and prevents him from taking the proper action. It is crucial that you begin to grasp how difficult it is for him to negotiate situations that evoke anger, sadness, or disappointment. What can seem to you like a small emotional brushfire feels to your child like a full-blown five-alarmer.

> *You need to understand how hard it is for your child to negotiate any situation that evokes anger, sadness, or disappointment. What seems like a small brushfire to you feels like a five-alarm fire to your child.*

Dysregulated people fall into three patterns of re-action when their emotions are stimulated. These groupings are relatively distinct, but notice that in each case the teens resort to self-injury when they find an emotion intolerable—either the initial emotion or a secondary one triggered by a reaction to the event. Over time a person may fit into more than one category.

Kids Who Lash Out

Alysa started her session with me by saying: "It happened again. My mother really pissed me off. We were at the mall and she wanted me to try on this sweater. She knows I hate it when she picks out clothes for me. I tried to be cool but she just kept insisting. Finally I just started screaming at her. People stared at me—I know I must have looked crazy, but I couldn't stop myself. Finally she just walked away. I felt horrible. I couldn't stand how awful I felt about losing it in the store with my mother. I went to the ladies' room and cut myself."

Alysa belongs to the group of kids who manage their dysregulation by lashing out at the people around them. Anybody can be a target when these kids begin to get revved up. They are quick-tempered and poor at expressing their anger effectively. Once their anger subsides, however, they often feel a great deal of shame about how they behaved. When their shame (a secondary emotion) becomes intolerable, they are likely to engage in self-injury.

Kids Who Act Impulsively

Mari and I had been working together in therapy for about 2 months when she told me about this phone conversation with her boyfriend: "He wasn't really being unreasonable. He was trying to tell me that we couldn't get to-gether on Friday night because his schedule at work had changed. It was automatic—I didn't even think about it. I just told him we were done and that I never wanted to see him again. He tried to apologize. I just don't know what I was thinking. Right after I hung up the phone on that idiot of a boy-friend, I was so depressed and pissed off, I just had to fix the way I was feeling. I marched straight upstairs and into the bathroom to use the razor on my arm."

When emotionally dysregulated, Mari and others like her are prone to impulsive actions like self-injury or substance use or making poor decisions about relationships. These are the people we often characterize as impulsive: they go from zero to 60 in a nanosecond, without even a faint notion of the consequence. Even when their initial impulsive act is not self-injury, after they have moved into action they may experience unbearable shame or self-loathing, similar to people who fly into rages. They're not out of the woods yet; these secondary emotions about their impulsive behavior may then lead them to self-injure.

Kids Who Feel Overwhelmed and Need to Soothe Themselves

Nora and I were speaking about her most recent episode of cutting, which oc-curred right after she and her boyfriend had yet another fight.

"He knew I was having a hard time and that I really needed him. How could he do this to me?" she complained. "He's the only person who can calm me down when I get like that."

"That must have been awful for you," I said. "Tell me all the feelings you were having in that moment."

"I don't know. I just felt like I was going to explode if I didn't get some relief," Nora replied, her eyes fixed on mine.

"When you get emotionally revved up, it seems it's hard for you to know just what it is that you feel," I suggested.

"I don't have to be upset not to know what I feel," Nora admitted. "I can never figure it out exactly."

Nora belongs to the third group, those who hurt themselves as a way of self-soothing. As with those adolescents in the other groups, the simpler paths to emotional regulation are not open to her. Nora could find no other way to release her emotions than to slice into her skin.

Where do you see your child among these descriptions? The better you understand these patterns, the more likely you'll be to know when to worry

---

1. Which of the three patterns of reaction (lashing out, acting impulsively, or needing to soothe) does your child tend to display?
2. What are the most common triggers that set off your teen's emotional dysregulation?
3. Typically, does your child have more trouble in the immediate aftermath of the emotion, or secondarily, as a response to feeling bad about how he or she behaved in reaction to it?

---

and move into action and when you'll just have to bear your regular level of parental anxiety.

EMOTIONAL ILLITERACY: WHAT DO I FEEL?

As I mentioned earlier, teens who are emotionally vulnerable often just don't know *what* they're feeling. All they know is that they can't stand it. Teens who can't identify or label their emotions are at a distinct disadvantage, one that has far-reaching implications. This trait can make it almost impossible for them to keep their behavior under control, to keep their friendships from becoming strained, to think clearly when their emotions start to rise, or to achieve a solid sense of identity. I'll talk more about this in the next chapter but, as you can see, emotional dysregulation can affect all aspects of your child's life. He will have difficulty communicating his needs (how can he get reassurance and comfort from you if he can't tell you that he's feeling extreme fear?). He will have a hard time believing his feelings are valid (if he's totally confused about what he's feeling, those feelings won't seem very trustworthy). And he will have trouble developing strategies for soothing himself or regulating his emotional reactions (how can he "talk himself down" when he has no idea what's bothering him so much?).

As we all know, each of our emotions can be experienced across a broad range of intensity. We can feel anger as anything from mild annoyance to murderous rage. Likewise, sadness runs

> *The inability to identify, label, and modulate their emotions brings enormous difficulty to these children in several key areas of behavior and communication, affecting everything from holding on to friendships to developing a solid sense of identity.*

the gamut from disappointment to deep grieving. In addition, each emotion can be thought of as having three components: (1) a feeling or sensation, (2) a cognitive element, and (3) a tendency toward certain actions. When we feel sad, for example, we may (1) have a sinking feeling or a sensation of a weight on our chest, (2) think about our troubles, and (3) feel like lying down. Recognizing these components—being "emotionally literate"—is essential for us to identify and accurately label our emotions and to determine what to do about them.

While our emotions can be felt across a range of intensity, there are really only a handful of fundamental emotions that we feel. In the following list, the first six emotions are sometimes referred to as the "pure emotions"—because they are more biologically based—while the last four are most likely learned. Furthermore, each of these emotions corresponds with a particular facial expression that cuts across cultures and eras. Wherever you go on this planet, you can "read" someone's expression and have a good idea of the corresponding feeling. Emotions are useful tools of communication—in fact, most of human communication is accomplished without words. Being emotionally literate is the key to this process.

The pure emotions are:

1. Anger
2. Sadness
3. Joy
4. Surprise
5. Fear
6. Disgust
7. Shame
8. Guilt
9. Envy
10. Jealousy

Inability to Ask for Help

Jack is a sensitive 16-year-old boy who has been cutting himself for about 18 months. He is very sympathetic and understanding when his friends have troubles, but he can't seem to turn that quality in on himself.

"I hate myself for feeling sad," he told me in one session. "It makes me feel like such a wimp. I wish I didn't have any feelings at all. They just make me feel crappy about myself."

Life is confusing enough for adolescents, but for those who don't know what they feel, it's exponentially more confusing. Kids who can't accurately label their feelings are left without an important blueprint to guide their actions. Instead, they experience a powerful and confusing inner state that feels unbearable. Their behavior becomes directed toward changing their inner state immediately rather than, for example, talking it out with another person or finding a safe strategy to help themselves calm down. What this boils down to is that these kids have great difficulty in asking for help and/or developing ways to help calm themselves down when they are upset, as Penelope's story illustrates.

> Kids who can't label their feelings have no blueprint for action. Instead of asking for help or developing ways to calm down, they've learned to do something that will change their powerful inner state immediately.

"Last night I had a wicked fight with my father. He can be such an idiot. Doesn't he know by now that he isn't helpful when I'm upset?" Penelope told me. "He heard me crying in my room after instant messaging with my best friend, who was being a jerk. He started asking me all these questions about how I was feeling. You know, am I angry or sad or worried? I know he was trying to be helpful and kind, but I didn't know what I was feeling and he was just making it worse. He wouldn't stop pestering me. Giving me all this advice about how I could solve the problem. I just started screaming at him to shut up! Finally he got really angry with me and stormed out of the room. I was so upset I just had to cut myself."

If Penelope had been able to identify her feelings and had some coping strategies at her fingertips that would lower the intensity of her feelings, she would have been much less likely to engage in self-harming behavior. Some simple, immediate solutions would have been to go jogging or to listen to some upbeat music or to take a bubble bath. While these strategies would not have solved her interpersonal problems, they might have helped her to regulate her feelings and calmed her down enough so that she could think clearly about what she wanted to do and maybe even tell her father what she was feeling.

Cooking Negative Feelings

Physiologically our feelings last a very short period of time and then dissipate on their own. In fact, to make our feelings last longer we have to keep doing whatever it is that evokes the feeling or keep thinking in a particular way about what generated the feeling. The kind of thinking that keeps negative feelings going is usually spiced with judgments about others or negative opinions about ourselves: a judgment about how unfair the situation is, or a feeling that there's something wrong with us for having the feeling in the first place, or that if I were a better person, I wouldn't feel this way.

For example, if your boss tries to blame you for something that wasn't your fault, in all likelihood you will experience some degree of anger. The feeling of anger will rapidly fade, however, once you stop thinking about what he did. But if you dwell on the situation, that anger will "cook" for a long time. When we cook our feelings long enough, they turn into moods. For example, for some kids journaling is a helpful strategy to help them calm down. For others, it just keeps them focused on what's troubling them. Consequently the more they write about a problem in a journal, the more they create a negative mood for themselves.

> *Any negative feeling, such as anger, will naturally fade after a short time. But dwelling on the situation that angered you, usually involving judging others or ourselves, will "cook" the anger long enough to turn it into a mood.*

When I asked Nora if she had any strategies besides cutting to help her calm down when she's emotionally revved up, she said: "Not really. Sometimes I try going to sleep or take some extra medications. But mostly I just stay feeling crappy, obsessing about what put me in such a bad mood. After a while I can't stand myself and I'm liable to pick a fight with whoever comes my way." Without the tools to soothe herself or to change her feelings, Nora can't help but lash out.

Modulating Emotion to Get Things Done

Being able to lower the intensity of our emotions and to avoid developing a "bad" mood as a misstep on the road to feeling calmer or needing to get tasks done is called *emotion modulation*. Anyone can practice enough to acquire the skill. If you're among those parents whose child has had trouble calming down after feeling sad or angry ever since she was little, here are some questions you might want to ask yourself to determine whether your child has problems with emotion modulation:

1. Does your child seem to get "stuck" in a bad mood that lingers well beyond the event that triggered it?
2. Does your child "demand" your help when he or she is upset, refusing help from any other adult? Yet at other times does he or she refuse help when you offer it?
3. Has it been extremely difficult for your child to make a transition to a new activity when he or she feels sad or angry?

This makes me think of a story from several years ago; when I was in my forties and I tried my hand at competitive cycling. I had the opportunity to train with a guy who was a bit older than I was but had been a former Olympian. I have to tell you that I put in more hours and miles per week on the bike than he did, and yet there was no way I could keep up with him. It wasn't a matter of practice and training; he was innately stronger on the bike than I was. In other words, he was just naturally better. Think about those things that have come relatively easily for you and those things that you had to work hard at mastering and you'll understand what I am getting at here.

> *Think about the skills that have come pretty easily to you in life compared to those you had to work hard for, and you can begin to see how hard it is for your child to regulate his or her emotions.*

It may be that people who are hard-wired to be emotionally reactive have to work harder at developing the capacity to regulate their emotions, but we just don't know for sure. Nor do we know what other innate variables come into play to make this easier or harder for a given person. What we do know is that most kids who engage in deliberate self-harm are at the emotionally reactive end of the emotional continuum. If they don't or can't modulate their emotions, they're more likely to make poor decisions, to fall prey to impulsive actions, and to be ineffective in their relationships.

To modulate his emotions, your child needs to activate the part of his brain that controls logical thinking and reasoning, that part of the brain that helps him reappraise his emotional situation, rather than the part that leaves him wallowing in the emotion. As you can see, emotion modulation skills are absolutely critical to our well-being.

Mood Dependency

In addition, being able to modulate our emotions makes it easier for us to sidestep an angry or depressive mood. Kids who lack this capacity tend to be mood-dependent—that is, their mood determines how effective they can be in carrying out their responsibilities and how they will experience any particular event. For example, if they're in a good mood, chances are they will be able to get their chores done and complete their school assignments or the long car ride to grandma's house will be pleasant. If they're in a bad mood, they may not be able to get anything done and neutral or even potentially pleasant events can get tainted by their negative emotions. If your child's behavior is mood-dependent, you may find it hard to understand that the trouble he's having has to do with his inability to modulate his emotions. After all, on the surface there's not much difference between mood-dependent behavior and sheer lack of motivation or willful disobedience. To make matters worse, he often won't be able to explain his behavior, except to say that at the time it seemed like a good idea. Skipping school to play video games, for example, may have seemed like a good idea to him at the time.

Ask yourself the questions in the accompanying box to help determine whether your child is mood-dependent:

---

1. Is there a big gap between what your child can do when he or she is relatively happy compared to what he or she can accomplish when a blue mood strikes?
2. Can your child harness himself or herself to choose the effective solution that the situation requires or does he or she take the easy path?
3. Can your child "let go"of his or her feelings to get chores done?

While we all find it easier to get our work done when we're feeling relatively calm, these kids experience a huge difference in their capacity to accomplish anything depending on whether they're calm or agitated. When they fall behind on life's requirements, they make their situation worse, increasing the likelihood that the bad mood will be extended.

What's Going On in the Brain?

Earlier I mentioned that kids who self-harm have more difficulty than the rest of us in calling on the part of the brain that controls logical thinking and reasoning. Researchers are beginning to study just how the brain operates when we modulate our emotions. Scientists can use functional MRIs to map the brain's activity as it works to solve particular problems. Here is a simplified version of what they have discovered about emotion modulation.

For the most part, emotions originate in a part of the brain called the amygdala. Depending on the situation, signals are sent from the amygdala to the prefrontal cortex, that part of the brain involved with reasoning. Here the brain works at evaluating what to do about the emotion. While there is nothing we can do to prevent ourselves from having a particular emotion, we *can* change how intensely and how long we experience it. Through the use of thought and logic, humans have developed several tried-and-true strategies to modulate their emotions.

Assuming we're in no imminent danger that requires an immediate response to our emotions—say, a ravenous lion is about to attack, in which case our fear would enable us to run for our lives—there are any number of strategies and skills we can use to modulate our emotions. In the following discussion, every emotion regulation strategy begins with accurately labeling and identifying our emotion. *All* the emotion regulation strategies are based on accepting and acknowledging what we feel. Emotion regulation is about (1) being willing to have the emotion, and then (2) working at modulating it. When we can't or won't accept our feelings, we inevitably make the situation worse either by cooking them or by impulsively moving into ineffective behavior.

Using Problem Solving to Modulate Emotions*

When we understand which situations are likely to produce intense negative reactions, any of us can use problem-solving skills either to avoid these situations or to craft some strategy that will lower the intensity of the feelings. For example, if you know that spending time with your angry and critical sister-in-law is going to rile you up, you might solve the problem by cutting your visits short or by meeting her in a public place that will make her less likely to go into a harangue.

This strategy might be useful in keeping the intensity of your feelings at a lower level, but not all situations will allow you to do this. Sometimes events happen that just get under your skin. In these moments you need some strategies to lower your emotional temperature. One example is to take an emotional time-out. Say you're at a party and someone makes a comment that really hurts your feelings. What do you do? The simplest thing would be to walk away and get absorbed in another conversation. Such a strategy may seem obvious to you, but would often be beyond the reach of your emotionally vulnerable child.

> *Simple problem-solving strategies that seem obvious to you may be beyond the reach of children who are emotionally vulnerable.*

LISA'S DRESS

Lisa and I were discussing the difficulty she'd had at a girlfriend's sleepover. We were trying to understand what had caused her to cut herself.

---

*The credit for much of what I outline in the following pages belongs to Marsha M. Linehan and her colleagues who developed DBT.

"I remember that Gina said something about my dress which, I don't know, upset me I guess," she explained. "All I remember is that I felt kind of spacey and maybe a little sad. I just stood there for a while and then I went into the bathroom and cut."

Lisa lacked two critical skills that prevented her from problem solving: (1) she couldn't accurately label and identify her emotions, and (2) she couldn't think clearly enough to find a better way to modulate her emotions.

Observing and Describing Emotions

It seems that in some cases simply identifying and accurately labeling our emotion can lessen its intensity. In essence, we just accept that how we feel at that moment is simply how it is. For example, the mere act of acknowledging that you are angry at your husband without either cooking it ("I can't believe he embarrassed me in front of his family again—he always does this") or trying to talk yourself out of it ("There's no reason for me to feel angry") may help in the process of modulating your emotion.

> *The simple act of acknowledging your negative emotion without "cooking" it or trying to talk yourself out of it can help you modulate the emotion.*

Several months after Lisa and I had discussed the trouble she'd had at her friend's sleepover, she came in to therapy and related this success: "My friends and I were at Marjorie's house yesterday and we were talking about what we were going to wear to the prom. I described my dress and Gina just made fun of it. This time I used some of the skills you've been going over with me and just observed and described to myself how I was feeling: insulted, hurt, mad. It really worked. I was still mad at Gina, but it just didn't seem so overwhelming to me."

Tell Yourself a Different Story

A second problem-solving strategy is to bring a process called "*reappraisal*" to our emotional experience. When we *reappraise*, we change our initial interpretation of the event that led to our emotion arising. Let's say you're at the grocery store and you notice that a friend whom you recently had over for dinner is coming down the aisle from the opposite direction. She passes you without a trace of acknowledgment. Almost immediately you are feeling hurt and angry. Your mind begins to weave a story to explain the situation: "I can't believe Danielle just ignored me like that. Well, clearly she didn't have a good time at dinner. Still, what kind of friend ignores you? Who does she think she is?" If you follow this path, you are certainly going to cook those negative feelings into a spicy emotional stew.

Suppose instead that you tell yourself a different story in response to your emotions: "Well, I'm surprised and hurt. I wonder why Danielle is so preoccupied that she didn't even see me. I hope everything is all right. I think I'll give her a call later and see what's going on."

In all likelihood this version of your story is going to decrease the intensity of your hurt and anger. You have accomplished this by reappraising or reinterpreting the event that evoked the feelings. Tell yourself a different story: it's a wonderful emotion regulation strategy and a handy tool when you don't know why something happened but you find yourself creating a story that makes you feel worse.

Acting in Opposition to How You Feel

I will have a great deal more to say about this powerful emotion regulation strategy in Chapter 8, but here is the short version. All our emotions, as I mentioned earlier, have an *action tendency* associated with them—that is, they make us want to take some kind of action. For example, sadness and depression often push us to lie down because we feel drained. Fear often makes us want to run away. Shame makes us want to hide or disappear. You can change the duration and intensity of these feelings by, first, acknowledging what you feel; second, deciding that you no longer want to feel it; and third, doing exactly the opposite of what the emotion is prompting you to do. If you're feeling blue and your whole being is saying "Get into bed and pull the covers up," you would instead throw yourself into some kind of physical activity.

Maureen, a 15-year-old DBT patient, paged me in crisis.

"I can't get out of bed. I am just too depressed, I have no energy, and I can't go see my cousins. They are all so perfect," she told me over the phone. "But if I don't go, my parents will kill me."

"Oh, man, you are between a rock and a hard place," I replied. "It seems like the better choice is to find a way to go, and that is going to take some real effort."

"I don't have the energy," she repeated.

"Yes, that is exactly what depression makes us feel. It saps us of our strength, and all we want to do is get into bed," I said.

"But I can't stay home!" Maureen exclaimed.

"Got it! I think it's time for opposite action to current emotion," I suggested. "Do you remember how this skill works?" I asked.

"Yes. I have to do the opposite action that my depression is telling me to do. Even though it feels like I have no energy, I have to get myself up and out of bed."

"Yes, that's right—and you have to commit 100% to the action. You can't do it halfway," I added.

"I think I just have to do this," she replied.

Distraction

Finally, we can use distraction as an emotion regulatory strategy. Like the other strategies, distraction usually starts by identifying and labeling your emotional experience. But if the experience is so intense that you can't clearly label the feeling, you can use distraction to lower the emotional intensity to try to get a better read on your emotional state. For example, it's late on a Friday afternoon and you open an e-mail from your boss criticizing your work. As you read it you realize that she lacks pertinent information that would change her point of view. Unfortunately she's left for the day and won't be back in the office until Tuesday. You notice that anger is rising up within you, but you know that you're going to be unable to resolve the situation until Tuesday. You decide that it would be a good idea to make yourself busy with activities and friends over the weekend. You distract yourself from your anger by picking up the phone and throwing yourself into making plans for the next couple of days.

ENVIRONMENTAL FACTORS: WHEN OUR BEST INTENTIONS FAIL

"Yesterday Celia came home from school and she was just a mess," her mother told me. "She and her best friend, Julia, had had a falling out. She has the same fight with this 'best friend' about 5 times a week, and it's getting a little old. I heard her up in her room slamming things around and cursing. It really unnerves me when she gets so emotional and I try not to think that she may hurt herself. I knew that she'd probably forgotten that she had SAT tutoring that day, and we were going to have to put a move on if we were going to be on time. I simply went upstairs and in a calm voice told her we needed to leave in 10 minutes. I should tell you that although I was calm on the outside, I was trying not to worry that this would turn into one of those several-hour meltdowns.

"Celia told me she wasn't going. Maybe I shouldn't have said it, but I reminded her how important this was for her future. I know she has bigger problems right now than getting into college, but I'm so worried she's going to make decisions now that will ruin her life. Anyway, that's when all hell broke loose. Celia started screaming that I didn't understand and all I was interested in was college. That did it for me. I told her that her friend Julia was a loser, and I couldn't understand how she didn't see that."

Does this sound familiar? Clearly the mom did her best in the beginning to keep the situation low key, which makes sense, given Celia's emotional state. What went wrong? Let's look a little more closely to see if we can figure out what Celia's mom could have done differently that might have prevented a meltdown.

Here's what we know: Celia is emotionally dysregulated, and her mom needs to get her to tutoring on time. We can speculate about a few other factors: Mom is losing patience with the repeated troubles in Celia's relationship with her friend, she's understandably put off by Celia's out-of-control behavior, and she's worried that her daughter will lose sight of her responsibility to go to SAT tutoring.

Here's what happened: Mom's strategy seems to have ignored her daughter's emotional distress and focused instead on the issue of getting out of the house on time. Why didn't that bring the desired results?

The central problem was a lack of validation. It's a common tactical error that we all make, and it can lead to all sorts of difficulties. To *validate* someone is to communicate that you understand that person's experience. You don't have to like it or agree with it; you just have to acknowledge it. When you don't validate, interpersonal communication is more likely to stall. Just imagine that a friend has

> With the best of intentions, someone may tell you not to let something bother you that is bothering you. We want the people who care about us to understand what we're feeling before they move on to how we can get over it.

hurt you, and your spouse tells you not to let it get to you because it's "no big deal." How well does that play? Even if ultimately it turns out not to be a big deal, you want your spouse to understand that it hurts right now.

Validating Your Child and Yourself

Celia's mom didn't validate Celia's emotional distress, and she seemed to invalidate her own worry through avoidance. (We need to validate ourselves, too. When we self-validate, we are acknowledging what we feel without avoidance or judgment.) It may have worked better had the exchange gone something like this: "So Julia did it again. I know she can really get under your skin. It must be hard to like someone who also can be so irritating. Anything I can do to help? No? Okay, then. As angry as you are, you probably forgot about tutoring."

"I'm not going."

"It's really hard to shift gears and think about tutoring when you feel so hurt and angry. That makes perfect sense. But this is a commitment and we need to leave in 10 minutes."

In my experience, invalidation generally stems from parents' reasonable and good intentions for their children. The terms *validation* and *invalidation* might sound condemning or critical, but please understand that I am in no way blaming you or saying that you're responsible for your children's troubles. After 30-plus years of working with children and parents, I have seen that the overwhelming majority of parents only want to be helpful to their kids. Kids who are extremely sensitive are a special parenting challenge. Please read the following sections as examples of how our best intentions can go south and what we can do to make things better. My only goal is to help you understand what might account for your best parenting efforts falling short.

There are different degrees of validation and invalidation. Kids who are emotionally reactive are probably more sensitive to even the mildest incidents of invalidation. So what may be no big deal for one child may be experienced as a very big deal for another. Hold on—it gets even more complicated: what may be experienced as mildly invalidating on one occasion could be felt as really invalidating on another if the child is emotionally charged up. Short of being candidates for sainthood, how can you validate in the midst of your own worry and your kids' emotional storms? In Chapters 6 and 7 I will have more to say about this, but for now here's the short course.

Three key factors will optimize your chances for success in those emotionally perilous moments. First, get very clear about your goal. In the earlier example, the goal was to get Celia to tutoring on time. Second, make sure to self-validate, and decide how you're going to manage your feelings. Again, in my example, Mom needed to honor her worry about Celia's future by acknowledging that this is how she felt, even though it wasn't going to be effective to give voice to it in light of the shorter term goal of getting Celia to tutoring. Finally, work at validating your child to help defuse the emotional crisis. Mom validated Celia when she expressed her understanding about her hurt and anger.

For your emotionally sensitive child not to become emotionally vulnerable, she may need extra help from you to learn emotion regulation skills. No one gave you a childrearing manual, and you may not know intuitively what she requires. Every since she was little, your child may have been more sensitive than others to life's hurts and disappointments. It's natural for you to have been downplaying her emotional response all along, or offering reassurance that things aren't as bad as she thinks they are. If your child seems to be having what you perceive to be an exaggerated response to a minor hurt, what parent wouldn't want to reassure him or her and try to put the problem into some more reasonable perspective?

This is a situation where parents' well-meaning intentions can backfire. Sometimes it's harder for parents to see their child's sensitivity during the elementary school years. Some parents tell me that they thought everything was right on track until adolescence, when suddenly it seemed like the wheels just came off and they were dealing with a totally different kid. My best guess is that some emotionally reactive kids have less trouble during middle childhood. The rules for behavior are clearer, and parents really can and do solve many of the child's difficulties. The new demands of the teen years—the biological changes, the emotional swings, the capacity for abstract thinking, and the broadening of possibilities in the social world—often present a rocky terrain for these teens to navigate.

> *Some parents tell me that they thought everything was right on track until adolescence, when suddenly it seemed like the wheels just came off and they were dealing with a totally different kid. The new demands of the teen years—hormonal and emotional shifts, a new capacity for abstract thinking, and the beckoning of a social world—often make things especially hard for emotionally vulnerable kids.*

KEISHA: VALIDATION AND INVALIDATION

"Keisha is just too sensitive!" her mom explained to me. "When she has a problem with a friend, it's like the end of the world for her. When I try to reassure her that I understand because I've had problems with my own friends, she just blows up. It's so awful for me when I'm trying so hard to help and she just pushes me away. Then I get hurt and angry and usually go to my room and cry and it just becomes a big mess."

"Yeah, and if you try to let her know that the whole thing is not such a big deal and give her some advice, she runs out of the room crying and screaming that you don't understand," added Keisha's dad. "That really frosts my socks, and I won't speak to her until she apologizes."

Keisha's parents' attempts to help with her troubles are eminently reasonable and clearly well intentioned. As any of us might do instinctively,
Mom acts reassuringly and Dad tries to help with problem solving. Clearly,
however, their attempts at being useful to their daughter fall short of the
mark. Is Keisha just an unreasonable person who revels in the drama of interpersonal conflict? Does she just not want to be comforted or to get the benefit
of parental advice, preferring to make a scene? Not likely. No one would
choose to live in such an emotionally distressed way and relish constant interpersonal turmoil.

There is another explanation for Keisha's behavior. Let's start by making
a couple of assumptions about her. First, let's assume that she was born with
an emotional system that is on the highly reactive end of the spectrum. Second, we will assume that she has not developed the skills that are required to
effectively regulate and modulate her emotions. Her parents' description
would seem to confirm that assumption. Consequently, we can consider
Keisha to be emotionally vulnerable.

As discussed, people who are emotionally vulnerable are usually emotionally reactive, and they also lack emotion regulation skills because they
haven't had sufficient modeling or validation about their emotional experience. In fact, we can get a glimpse into some possible reasons why Keisha has
not learned to regulate her emotions. Before we do that, however, let's revisit
the concept of validation and introduce its opposite, invalidation.

Remember that when we validate another person, we are simply communicating that we understand his or her current experience and how, under
the circumstances, it makes sense. We just accept the other person's experience as it is, without making a judgment and without offering a solution.
Problem solving, which of course is terribly important, can be thought of as
the opposite of validation. When we are invalidating, our communication to
the other person is that his or her current experience is not justified; it's exaggerated or inaccurate under the cir-
cumstances. We all invalidate one
another from time to time, so it becomes a problem only when it's a frequent aspect of family communication. Invalidation can also occur
outside the family and be a real prob-

> *As important as problem solving
> is, it runs counter to validation,
> in which we want to accept the
> person's experience just as it is.*

lem for a child. A family may be quite validating of their sensitive child, who
then enters a school environment that may be such a mismatch that the child
feels harshly misunderstood and judged.

For example, a very sensitive child may feel continually invalidated in a regimented traditional school setting in which academic results are valued over personal growth. Another example of invalidation is bullying by other children when it's not effectively addressed by the adults in charge. This is especially true when the adults expect the child to be more assertive in stopping the bullying or tell the child to stop letting it bother him so much.

Validation is a key task of parenting. When we validate our children, we are teaching them how to accurately label their inner experiences and to trust those experiences and use them to self-validate and effectively problem solve. When we invalidate our children, of course, we create just the opposite situation. We teach them that what they feel is inaccurate or inappropriate to the situation. Here are two examples of parental invalidation:

1. "You shouldn't be hurt by your friend; you should be angry that he treated you that way."
2. "So you didn't get invited to the party. That's no big deal—after all, these kids hardly know you."

In both examples the intention of the parent is to be helpful, but you can see how the response invalidates the child's experience.

Helping children problem-solve in the moment and helping them anticipate problems and plan for the future is another important task of parenting. When it comes to this task there are two common pitfalls that lead to invalidation and compromise the child's effectively learning to problem-solve.

Problem Solving Too Early

The first error is to problem-solve *before* validating. It's a very easy trap to fall into. After all, you just want to resolve whatever problem is causing your child so much pain. You can probably already see that Keisha's father succumbed to it when he told Keisha that her problem with her friend was no big deal and immediately tried to give her advice.

Letting Your Own Bigger Worries Get in the Way

The second problem occurs when parents are having difficulty tolerating their own worries about their children's capacity to effectively problem-solve. Celia's mom provides a good example. In the face of her daughter's emotional distress, she understandably began to worry about what Celia's lack of commitment to the SAT tutoring might portend. Introducing her own (perfectly reasonable) worry into the situation invalidates her daughter's current experience. Celia is also the kind of kid who is hypersensitive to other's emotions, particularly those of her parents—from whom she wants approval, even if she won't admit it. Her mother's worry about her overwhelms her and makes her worry about herself at a time when she can't handle any more emotional input.

As you can see, the kicker is that you can be invalidating even when your intentions are to be helpful. There are degrees of invalidation that run from the well-intentioned parent who's just trying to be helpful to a distressed child, all the way to child abuse. Human beings just seem to do better when we're understood and tend to get more emotionally dysregulated when we're not. When we're misunderstood we often work hard at getting the understanding that we need. How skillful we are at this will be part of our story.

Let's take a closer look at the ways each of Keisha's parents respond to their daughter. Please keep in mind that these are reasonable parents struggling to find a way to be helpful to their child.

Why Reassurance Isn't Validating

The first thing we notice is that Mom seems to rely on two strategies to be helpful. The first strategy is reassurance; the second is to bring her own history into the discussion as a way of letting Keisha know that she understands. Clearly these two seemingly reasonable strategies don't work. Why not?

When you are emotionally revved up and someone tells you that everything is going to be okay, your feeling may be that the person can't possibly appreciate the magnitude of the problem. Consequently, rather than feeling understood and reassured, you're likely to feel invalidated. Reassurance is a strategy that is often effective with younger children who are more willing to be dependent on an adult's point of view. The preschooler who is nervous about a play date with a new friend is likely to be calmed down by a parent who reassures her that she'll be fine. Not so for the teenager whose parent says the same thing about another friend's hurtful comment.

Adolescents are often less willing than young children to buy into an adult's viewpoint. Therefore they're less likely to be reassured just because you tell them everything is going to be all right.

Naturally, we rely on strategies that have worked for us in the past; therefore parents sometimes offer up reassurance just because it used to work. Once your child reaches adolescence, however, she has a strong instinct to be her own person and rely less on you. In addition, during adolescence the brain becomes capable of process-ing more abstract ideas. Since the world is no longer so easy to understand, your simple reassurance is experienced by your teen as unrealistic.

Why Saying "I've Been There" Isn't Validating

Keisha's mom also tries to let her know that she understands how Keisha feels by bringing in examples from her own life. Again, this appears reasonable—Keisha's mom is looking for common ground. The hope is that Keisha would feel her mom has some credibility because she too has struggled with friend-ships. Despite all the right intentions, the effect of Mom's behavior is to make Keisha feel misunderstood.

What went wrong?

When we try to let someone know that we understand his or her situa-tion by bringing in examples from our own lives, we run the risk of shifting the focus toward ourselves and away from the person in need. Furthermore, it is the exceptional adolescent who is going to believe that her parents' situa-tion "back in the day" can have any relevance to her own. It's only likely to make your child feel more misunderstood, not less.

Why Putting Things into Perspective Isn't Validating

Let's turn our attention now to Keisha's dad. He enters the fray by trying to help put Keisha's difficulties into a more reasonable perspective. While he may be on to something, this approach is almost guaranteed to be invalidat-ing. Why? Although it is certainly not his intention, by telling his daughter that she is making too big a deal of something, especially when she is dysregulated, he's invalidating her experience. Please remember that he is dealing with an emotionally distressed teenager, not someone who is cur-rently functioning rationally or fully in charge of her reactions.

Why the Best Advice Given Too Soon Isn't Validating

Then Dad compounds his mistake by offering unsolicited advice to the very person he has just invalidated. What is the chance Keisha is going to be grateful for his words of wisdom? Zero! The real shame here is that his advice might be right on the money. For whatever the reason—maybe it's a design flaw—people are more willing to accept advice after they feel they've been understood. Very often an adolescent I have been treating will tell me a story about a parent's attempts at problem solving before validating. Later in the therapy I'll ask, "With the distance you have now, how would you assess the advice?" Invariably, he or she tells me that the advice was pretty good, but the timing was terrible.

Master Class: You Need to Model Emotion Regulation Skills

I hope you can begin to see the subtle ways invalidation works. When it's a pervasive part of the interaction between parent and child, it becomes very difficult for the child to learn to identify and to trust the accuracy of his or her emotional experience. When this happens children are prone to being pushed around by their emotions rather than being competent at managing them. In later chapters I'll give you some suggestions about how to get better at validation. For now, be warned about reassurance; stay away from bringing in your own history (unless it's asked for); and make sure you have validated before moving into problem solving. But wait—there's more!

Both of Keisha's parents report having very strong emotional responses to their daughter's seemingly unreasonable behavior. This, of course, is perfectly understandable. They're trying their best to be helpful and the whole thing is blowing up right in their faces. How they manage their own emotional turmoil, however, is another potential problem. To stay on track, emotionally reactive kids need more validation than other kids, and they need parents who can model effective emotion regulation skills. I understand that at times this is certainly easier said than done! My own kids will tell you that I have lost my temper with them too. Keisha's parents are not helping the situation either by becoming outwardly dysregulated or by withdrawing into an icy silence. Their daughter really needs her parents, most of the time, to show her by their own behavior that emotions can be regulated to improve interpersonal relationships and attain a balanced sense of well-being. Please read Chapter 7 to see whether you need to work on this.

The Snowball Effect of Invalidation

When an emotionally reactive child meets an invalidating environment, the climate is just right for a "perfect storm" of trouble. The interaction of the two has a synergistic effect, like a snowball going downhill that just keeps picking up speed as it builds upon itself. This snowball effect generally follows two distinct patterns. The first is distinguished by an escalation of the child's behavior in a desperate attempt to be understood. Here is a story that I think brings this concept home.

Desperate to Be Heard: Floyd and the Farmer

One summer during my college years I hitchhiked through Europe with my brother and a college friend named Floyd. Floyd spoke a little French but not enough to get by. Soon after we arrived in France we were picked up by a farmer, and we attempted to communicate to him where we were headed. Floyd started using his French but couldn't make himself understood. The farmer became increasingly frustrated with him. Floyd responded by speaking louder, as if he would be better understood at a higher volume. When it was clear that the farmer still had no idea what Floyd was saying, Floyd spoke even louder and began to introduce English words into the mix (albeit with a French accent). It was chaos. The farmer just dropped us off in the nearest town.

I use this story as a metaphor for the transactional nature between an emotionally reactive child and an invalidating environment. When a child feels invalidated, her emotions run high and she redoubles her efforts to be understood. Unfortunately, emotionally vulnerable kids are not skilled in this regard and, like Floyd, usually just raise the decibel level rather than figuring out a way to express what they need. Naturally, the reaction from people around them—the environmental response—will be aimed at the "loud" behavior and not at the emotional need behind it. Consequently the child feels more invalidated, which intensifies her emotional dysregulation. Now overwhelmed with intense feelings and lacking regulation skills, the child is prone to self-injure. This transactional cycle takes on a life of its own, and over time it becomes a stable if dysfunctional communication pattern.

The Silent Treatment

In the second pattern, the child's sense of being misunderstood and the accompanying hurt go underground as she becomes increasingly silent and withdrawn. Family members may then increase their efforts to get the child to reveal herself, which meets with only more silence. The child has given up on being understood and just retreats into silence and phony compliance with parental expectations. On the inside, however, she is still struggling to manage her emotional turmoil. Frequently these are the children who have learned to mask their feelings. Often the parents don't even suspect that the child is in trouble until they discover that he or she has been self-harming.

Each of these patterns represents a different response to feeling misunderstood and the emotional dysregulation that follows. As we will see, the self-harm is most often aimed at regaining emotional balance.

Does your child fit the pattern of using self-harm to manage painful emotions?

---

1. Is your child at the emotionally reactive end of the continuum?
2. Are you able to determine whether he or she is emotionally vulnerable and lacking in the skills required to modulate emotion?
3. Does your child seem to go from one emotional crisis to another? Or is he or she the kind of child who masks feelings?
4. Think about your typical responses to your teen's emotional distress. Do you tend to unwittingly make things worse? It's important to grasp the concept of how the ingredients of emotional vulnerability and invalidation snowball into an increased level of emotional dysregulation.

If the answers to most of these questions is yes, then in all likelihood your child is using deliberate self-harm as a way of managing emotional distress. In the next chapter we'll look more closely at the variety of ways kids use self-harm to manage their emotions, as well as at some self-harming behavior that is *not* in the service of emotional regulation.

3

how does hurting themselves make some kids feel better?

The preceding chapter helped you understand the factors that predispose children to hurting themselves. But what does self-injury actually accomplish? This chapter helps you recognize the problems your child is trying to solve through deliberate self-harm, which will make it easier for you to select and assess the proper therapy.

REGAINING EMOTIONAL BALANCE

"I did it again," Lea whispered into the phone. "It really chilled me out. I kind of felt calm, like things were going to be okay. The feeling didn't last too long, but at least I stopped feeling crazy on the inside."

"Yeah, I know what you mean," replied her friend Jonathan. "I know I shouldn't do it either, but it's my body and it really does work when you feel that way."

It's hard for us to comprehend how hurting yourself can produce a feeling of calmness, but for certain emotionally overwhelmed individuals it does. We just don't know what differentiates those people for whom deliberate self-harm works as a self-soothing mechanism from those for whom it doesn't. Nor do we know exactly why and how it works to soothe and calm kids. At this point all we can say is that the mechanism is probably a combination of biological and some as yet unspecified psychological factors.

It is important that you understand the degree to which your teen feels emotionally overwhelmed and out of control. While some of these kids are pretty good at keeping their level of distress hidden, inside they are a whirl-wind of emotional chaos. If parents can't tell when their kids are emotionally revved, the self-harm may look like an impulsive act that comes out of the blue. While it might be impulsive, it certainly didn't come out of the blue.

Marissa was feeling deeply hurt by her friends, whom she felt did not in-clude her in the discussion at lunch. To make the day worse, she got a C– on an English paper on which she thought she had done well. On the way home, she phoned her best friend for some support.

"Hey, what's up?" asked Kristin in a cheerful voice.

"Nothing. I'm just having a crappy day," Marissa replied

"That sucks!" Kristin said. "What are you doing later? I'm going to chill with Sara. Hey, I'm getting another call. I'll call you back."

Click! The line went silent.

When Marissa's mom described that evening to me later, she said: "I kind of knew that something might be wrong when Marissa came home from school. She was a little quieter than usual, but I just thought she might be tired. When I asked her how she was, she just said 'fine' and went upstairs to her room. When she came down for dinner, she was in a much better mood. During dinner I noticed the blood on her sleeve."

When children hide their distress, their parents are in an especially diffi-cult position. There is a natural tendency on the parents' part to become more vigilant, which the child customarily experiences as intrusive and so he or she may in response become even more secretive. In addition there is a natural tendency for adolescents to seek privacy. On the other hand, it's aw-fully difficult for a parent to stand by and do nothing. Parents who find them-selves in this dilemma have to negotiate the foggy waters between the shoals of harmful secrecy and the open channel of age-appropriate privacy. We will examine how to navigate these waters in Chapter 6.

"It took us a long time to figure out when we could trust Candice with some privacy and when she needed us to be more attentive. We started to be able to read the subtle signs of trouble and how to gently offer our help. It didn't always work, but when it did it was good. For example, we slowly were able to distinguish the buzzwords that let us know she was having trouble."

Like Candice, most kids describe the sense of "going crazy" with intense emotions. They wish they could "jump out of their skins" to escape the emo-tional pain: "It's like I'm on emotional fire. I can't think straight and feel all panicky on the inside. Nothing makes sense and I just have to end this horri-ble feeling." Another patient told me: "When I get what you call 'emotionally dysregulated,' I'm just a mess. Inside I am overwhelmed with intense feelings, and on the outside I am screaming and crying at the same time."

As you've learned, these kids often can't accurately label their feelings. They experience their emotions as an intense hodgepodge of inner sensations. If in these moments of inner turbulence you attempt to get a clear reading of what your child is experiencing, you're likely to get a reaction that's a combination of anger and tears. The problem is that these children really do experience emotions more deeply and more quickly than the rest of us, and they have real trouble bringing themselves back from an emotional event. Without the capacity to modulate their emotions they, like a person who is drowning, flail about in an emotional panic, reaching for something to save them. Deliberate self-harm can become the flimsy but functional life preserver that resolves their inner turmoil.

> *Like someone who's drowning, people who can't modulate their emotions flail about and reach for something to save them. Their self-harming behavior is the only life preserver they can find.*

Self-Injury as Painkiller

Immediately following self-injury these children experience a period of calmness and relief. How long this sense of relief lasts differs for every child and even from episode to episode. It can last anywhere from a few short minutes to several days. When people feel as desperate as these kids do, getting even a moment's relief feels like a gulp of cool water on a parched throat.

Diminishing Returns

Ruth has been cutting herself at least three times a week for the past 2 years. The following conversation occurred in our first meeting.

"So, Ruth, you're pretty clear that cutting helps you regain some emotional relief when you are really upset," I said. "Have you noticed that you have to cut more frequently in each episode of self-harm to get relief?" I asked.

"Yeah, it used to be that I could cut once and I would feel calm. Now I have to cut 10 or 15 times to get the same feeling," she replied.

Like someone who is addicted to opiates, Ruth is one of those kids who need to keep upping the dosage to get the same result. In all likelihood there is a biological basis for this phenomenon. In moments of self-injury the body releases certain chemicals (that are, in fact, similar to opiates) as a way of helping to manage the tissue damage and pain. Some children's bodies seem to adapt to the initial levels of these chemicals. When this happens, they need to injure more frequently in order to attain the same sense of calmness.

> *The act of self-injury releases chemicals into the body—not unlike what using opiates would do—to help manage the tissue damage and pain. Some teens' bodies adapt to these chemicals, and they need to injure themselves more often to reach the same state of calm.*

How and why deliberate self-harm works this way for some kids and not others is not clearly understood. In both situations the relief most likely comes from the opiate-like substances that are released at the time of injury. We all have different responses to drugs; for example, some people have a low tolerance for alcohol, while others can drink a much larger quantity before they get intoxicated. While there are several different influences that contribute to a person's "drug of choice," body chemistry is certainly one important factor.

Is your child self-injuring to relieve emotional pain?

1. Does she seem to escalate the harm to herself with each successive incident?
2. Does the self-injury seem addictive?
3. Are there multiple wounds when she self-injures?

Self-Injury as Suicide Prevention

"When I feel so down and hopeless that suicide seems like a reasonable way out, I turn to cutting," Brad told me. "I don't want to kill myself, and I get really scared when I start thinking that way. I know cutting will take the edge off."

A small number of kids, like Brad, turn to self-injury as a kind of suicide prevention strategy. These are a subset of children who are struggling with both suicidal preoccupations and emotional vulnerability. They're trying to escape from the intense fear and anxiety that often accompany suicidal ideation. In a desperate attempt to end the disturbing preoccupation, they turn to deliberate self-harm.

These children are struggling to manage both emotional dysregulation and thoughts and feelings about suicide. They may be at higher risk for suicide. While it is always important for parents to obtain a careful assessment of their children's deliberate self-harm, it's especially critical for this subgroup of kids to be identified and undergo an ongoing risk assessment as part of their treatment.

Is your child self-injuring as a way to stave off suicide? (See also the box on page 23 in Chapter 1.)

1. Does he or she ever talk of suicide?
2. Has your child experienced a recent loss?
3. Has there been a recent suicide in the community?

Self-Injuring to Feel Alive

"I just couldn't take it anymore. I felt dead on the inside. You know, numb and empty," Jill complained. "I stopped feeling part of the world—it was kind of spooky. I felt like I was a zombie."

"How did cutting yourself change that?" I asked, anticipating her answer.

"I don't really know, but as soon as I made the first cut and saw the blood, I felt alive again."

To someone who feels dead or numb on the inside, life feels devoid of pleasure. It's as if everyone around him or her is living in a world of Technicolor and his or her life is in black and white. Each day is drudgery. In a way it's just the other side of the coin of emotional dysregulation: instead of overflowing with emotion, these kids feel none at all. It's not a state of being emotionally cold, but of being empty. To kids in this state, the world around them has an unreal quality to it; they feel more like a *spectator* of life than a *participant* in life. It feels as if they have lead weights on their feet—every step is a Herculean effort. There is often an overwhelming sense of aloneness. When our emotions are not available to us, our experience has a sterile, bland quality to it. Nothing seems to have much value, so it's difficult to hold on to goals.

> *When our emotions are unavailable to us, we feel numb and alone. Our lives feel sterile and bland, as if everyone else's life were in Technicolor and ours was in black and white.*

Our emotions are an extremely important source of information about how we are experiencing ourselves and the world around us. When this mirror is unavailable to us, we're prone to making poor and impulsive decisions about how to negotiate life's many challenges. Under these conditions we're likely to act in ways that are self-defeating and self-limiting at best, and po-tentially dangerous at worst.

As you can imagine, it's difficult to be in this state for any length of time. At some point it becomes more than a person can bear, and some effort be-comes directed toward changing this state of affairs. All too often a child who is contending with this experience moves quickly into behaviors that are in the service of ending the numbness in the short run but that often lead to more problems over the long haul. An indiscriminate sexual encounter or turning to drugs and alcohol can end the deadness, but even these poor solu-tions require some planning and access. Deliberate self-harm, unfortunately, can be done quickly, privately, and easily. Like Jill, kids who are struggling to end the deadness and numbness often report that they need to see blood be-fore they get relief from this awful state. It's almost as if seeing the blood con-firms that they're alive.

Often these children vacillate between feeling an inner numbness and feeling a deep and powerful sense of self-hatred. Many of them have endured the painful and confusing trauma of sexual abuse. So whenever the self-injury appears to be in the service of ending an adolescent's inner numbness, the adults in his or her life must at least consider whether there may have been a history of abuse. Some research suggests that victims of early sexual trauma may be prone to more severe self-injurious behavior. This has certainly been my clinical expe-rience.

> *Teens who resort to self-injury to end the feeling of inner deadness often vacillate between feeling emotionally numb and feeling a profound sense of self-hatred. Many of them have been victims of sexual abuse.*

This relatively small, but very worrisome, group of kids also is at higher risk for attempting suicide. One tragic consequence of early trauma is the child's belief that what happened was his or her fault. The legacy of this misguided belief is of-ten intense contempt and self-loathing. For these children, self-injury can func-tion as a self-soothing strategy and/or as an expression of deep-rooted self-hatred. When it is the latter, they literally attack their bodies as a way to punish themselves and to resolve the guilt and shame they experience for their imag-ined complicity in the sexual abuse.

Self-Injuring to Counter Feelings of Invisibility

"Sometimes I think they don't even know I exist or who I really am. They talk about me as though I wasn't standing right there. I hate it! Don't they know I have feelings too?" Lindsey complained.

Is your child self-injuring to feel alive again?

1. Does your child seem to be going through most of his or her days in a state of drudgery and emptiness?
2. Has your child ever claimed to have felt better as soon as he or she drew blood?
3. Was your child sexually abused? Do you need to investigate whether this is the case?

"You must feel kind of invisible when that happens," I said.

"Yeah, it's awful. It's like I just don't count for anything. Like I'm not that important even to my parents," she said between sobs. "I know it's the wrong thing to do, but when I cut myself they notice me and I feel like they see me and I feel real again."

Most of us at one time or another have been in a situation in which we have felt ignored, as if those around us didn't even notice our existence. It's an uncomfortable moment that can bring on intense emotions. Our options are to flee the situation or to do something that gets us noticed. The subset of children who self-harm and feel invisible usually don't want to be the center of attention or to feel jealous of the attention others are receiving. (Remember that only about 2 in 50 kids self-injures to get noticed.) They just want to stop the feeling of being invisible, of disappearing into the void.

Rather than being self-centered and taking dramatic steps to hog the spotlight, these kids feel unnoticed in their own families. This situation generally comes about when the child has the feeling of being ignored in her family. In my experience parents have not deliberately, or in some cases even unwittingly, overlooked their child. Instead, due to her innate sensitivity, she may need more affirmation than any parent could reasonably be expected to perceive. I have found that these children are often reticent about expressing their thoughts and feelings. Frequently their parents have a tough time understanding, and therefore tolerating, their kids' inability to articulate their thoughts and feelings. What ends up happening is that the parents fill in the gaps and thereby create a persona for their child. They then respond to the persona rather than to the real kid. Of course, the child complicates things by not correcting the parents' misperceptions.

> *Children who feel invisible may need more affirmation than parents could ever realize. They don't want to be the center of attention; they just need to stop the sense that they're disappearing into the void.*

"They say they know me and understand me, but all they know is how they want me to be, not how I really am," Lindsey continued. "Sometimes when they're talking about me, it sounds like they're describing a stranger. I wish I could tell them how I really feel. I'm too afraid they would be disappointed."

It's not unusual for these adolescents to begin to wonder whether they'll ever fit in and whether their parents value them. These kids rarely give voice to their concern, so their parents usually remain in the dark about these worries. The parents can find themselves in a no-win situation when their child resorts to deliberate self-injury: If they respond to the behavior with a fair amount of attention and soothing, they run the risk of reinforcing deliberate self-harm and at the same time confirming their own view that the self-injury is all about being at center stage. If, however, they respond with anger or even a more neutral position, that's likely to confirm the child's view

> One approach may sound odd or cold, but can be very effective: Pretend you are a loving anthropologist and adopt an attitude of patient curiosity.

of not being "seen" or understood. One way out of this dilemma is for parents to adopt an attitude of patient curiosity. Rather than push their kids to define themselves, parents can remain open and curious about their child. I sometimes describe this to parents as adopting the stance of a loving and caring anthropologist who is interested in studying a foreign culture.

Is your child self-injuring to counter feelings of invisibility?

1. Does your child have a lot of difficulty stating his or her thoughts and feelings?
2. Does your child's reticence extend so far that you often feed him or her the responses you think he or she should be giving you?
3. Does your child frequently complain of feeling misunderstood?

Self-Injury as Avoidance

"I just couldn't do it," Mona said. "There was no way I could get up in front of that class and make a speech. I just get so nervous. I'm sure I would have looked like a big loser. I'm not like the other kids in my class."

"A lot of people get really anxious in those kinds of situations," I replied. "It can be very tough for some folks to speak in front of people."

"I don't think you understand," Mona said slowly. "Just *thinking* about a situation like that makes me so tense that I just want to die. I was so scared and nervous the night before, I couldn't sleep—and nobody seemed to understand."

"I think I get it. You were feeling really desperate and trapped," I offered.

"Exactly. I had to do something, and cutting myself was the only thing I could think of. When my parents found out, they called my doctor and she told them to take me to the hospital. That was a real pain, but it was better than having to make my class presentation."

A small fraction of the kids who self-injure do so as a way to avoid situations with expectations they feel they can't manage. For these kids, certain upcoming events are so fraught with anxiety that self-injury seems to be the only way out. What differentiates these children from kids who use a stomachache or other feigned illness as an avoidance strategy is the degree of guilt and self-loathing they feel. When we avoid something, we usually experience mild or moderate guilt; we know we're doing the wrong thing, but we can tolerate our misstep. Kids whose avoidance takes the form of self-harm are in a different category altogether: their avoidance confirms their sense of weakness; it raises their level of self-loathing; and in combination with their anxiety, it produces an emotional experience that overwhelms them.

> The difference between the child who self-injures and the child who fakes a stomachache to avoid an event is the extreme guilt and self-loathing the self-injurer feels.

"It's just so hard to explain what happens for me," Mona continued. "I start to get really nervous about what I have to do. Then I start telling myself that there's nothing to be nervous about, which I think only makes it worse because I still feel anxious. That's when I start telling myself that I'm such a loser."

While the self-injury probably does calm the child's anxiety, its primary function is to help the teen avoid situations that he or she anticipates with intense dread. If you think your child falls into this category, it may be useful to get a consultation around treatment for anxiety in addition to therapy for self-injury.

MANAGING DISTURBING THOUGHTS: PSYCHOTIC ILLNESS AND OBSESSIVE–COMPULSIVE DISORDER

Two or more psychiatric conditions can exist in the same person at the same time. So sometimes self-injury is one aspect of other psychological problems,

Is your child self-injuring as an avoidance strategy?

1. Do you find that your child self-injures when you know he or she is anxious about an event in the near future?
2. After the injury, does your child focus on how it precludes his or her having to attend, perform, or otherwise be engaged in something he or she has been dreading?
3. Is your child generally anxious and does he or she seem to worry excessively about seemingly small matters?

problems that have less to do with managing emotional dysregulation than with managing disturbing thoughts. (Sometimes children with posttraumatic stress disorder, or PTSD, self-injure to avoid the intrusive memories called *flashbacks*, but since these flashbacks are almost always accompanied by the dysregulated emotions or feelings of emptiness I've already discussed, I won't address PTSD separately here.) I include here a brief description of two conditions that can coexist with self-injury just to complete the picture of deliberate self-harm. These children generally need a therapy other than the DBT that I'll discuss in Part II. It is very important that you obtain a thorough diagnostic assessment to help you understand the way self-injury fits into your child's current troubles.

NINA: HEARING VOICES

Nina walked into my office and slipped quickly into the chair across from me. Her face was nearly expressionless, giving no clue to what she might be feeling. I attempted to make some small talk to break the ice, but I only got one-word responses for my efforts.

"I understand that you've been hurting yourself. I hope that you'll be willing to talk with me about that for a few minutes," I said.

Nina only nodded her head in reply.

"I've spoken with many, many kids who have self-injured, and this is what I've learned from them. Some kids deliberately hurt themselves as a way of managing intense and overwhelming emotions. Other kids have told me that they hurt themselves when they feel numb and empty and that feeling becomes intolerable for them. Finally, some kids hurt themselves because the voices in their head tell them to do so. Do you think you fit into any of those categories?" I asked.

"The last one," Nina said softly.

Some children who have a major mental illness (bipolar disorder, schizophrenia, or schizoaffective disorder) experience auditory hallucinations—voices that "command" them to self-injure. While all psychological difficulties are due to an interaction of biological process and environmental influences (e.g., family, society), these conditions are probably more biologically than environmentally based. Frequently the "voices" are of a harsh and critical nature and demand that the children injure themselves as punishment. The child's brain processes these "voices" the same way it would process anything else he or she were to hear, and it can be very frightening. The "voices" seem very real to these kids and they may feel compelled to comply with their demands.

> *To kids who hear voices, they are very real. They may feel compelled to do what the voices tell them.*

While psychiatric medications can have some troublesome side effects (such as weight gain or slowed thinking), they can be very effective in treating hallucinations of this type. If you suspect that your child's deliberate self-harm is due to such "command hallucinations," the first order of business is a complete psychiatric evaluation that includes a psychopharmacological consultation, neuropsychological testing, and a thorough medical workup.

ROBIN: OBSESSIVE–COMPULSIVE DISORDER

When Robin walked into my office, the first thing I noticed were the bright red marks on her arms and legs. It was immediately clear that she had been picking at herself and that she was not allowing the wounds to heal. After a few minutes of chat we got down to business.

> *Obsessive–compulsive disorder can make you feel like a slave to the demand to get things "just right."*

"I couldn't help but notice the marks on your arms and legs. What is going on for you?" I asked.

"It's kind of crazy, I know, but once I start to pick at myself, I can't stop. I get this idea in my head that I just have to get it perfect. I kind of get lost in what I'm doing—I can spend hours in the bathroom looking in the mirror and picking at myself. It frightens me that I have no control over what I'm doing," Robin said as tears filled her eyes.

"Is it like you are a slave to the idea that you have to get it just right?" I wondered.

"Exactly!"

People with obsessive-compulsive disorder get fixated on an idea and often have to gratify that idea through compulsive and repetitive behavior. The very notion of not allowing themselves to engage in the behavior produces a sense of extreme dread and worry. For some children the compulsive behavior may take up hours of their time and compromise their ability to get their schoolwork done, or it may interfere with having a normal social life.

One kind of compulsive or ritualistic behavior is skin picking. As Robin explained, once these children begin the ritual, it's extremely difficult for them to stop. Frequently what drives the child's ritualistic behavior is some frightening idea that is accompanied by a powerful sense of dread. For example, she may feel that if she doesn't engage in the behavior, something awful will happen to a loved one.

Obsessive–compulsive disorder is more of a biologically based illness than a psychological disturbance caused by the interaction between the child and the environment. If your child's self-injury seems to follow this pattern, then a combination of cognitive-behavioral therapy and medication would be the best course of treatment.

Understanding the functions that deliberate self-harm serves for your child will help you and your child's mental health practitioner figure out which problems to target in treatment and which skills your child lacks for dealing with painful emotions and solving problems. I listed those emotion modulation strategies in Chapter 2. A major goal of therapy should be to help your child acquire those skills so that self-injury no longer performs a necessary function. (I'll show you later in the book how you can help your child learn better ways to handle emotion, particularly by offering the validation that your child needs to begin to understand and trust his or her emotions.)

The Importance of a Comprehensive Psychiatric Assessment

If your child is engaging in self-injury, your first step should be to obtain a thorough psychiatric assessment, for the following reasons.

Identifying Other Psychological Problems

As we've seen, self-injurious behavior can co-occur with other psychological problems such as auditory hallucinations or obsessive–compulsive disorder. Researchers have discovered that adolescents who engage in deliberate self-harm fall into a wide spectrum of diagnostic categories, from mood disorders (e.g., depression) to various forms of conduct disorders and personality disorders. One of the benefits of a thorough assessment is that it should help you determine whether your child is struggling with other problems.

Preventing Unaddressed Self-Injury from Leading to Suicidality

Second, there is a clear link between self-injurious behavior and suicidal behavior. No, I am not contradicting the points about suicide that I've made so far. Kids who harm themselves in the ways I've been describing are not doing it to try to end their lives, and they can almost always make a clear distinction between using self-injury to perform one of the functions I've described and trying to end their lives. A thorough assessment can determine whether your child is engaging in self-injury to soothe emotional distress or is suicidal.

But you should also know that helping your child stop injuring himself may prevent him from becoming suicidal in the future. It is not my intention to be unnecessarily alarming, but I want you to have the facts as we understand them in this moment. Some current research on the relation between nonsuicidal self-injury (i.e., deliberate self-harm that is used to control emotions) and suicide attempts indicates the following:

1. The longer someone engages in deliberate self-harm, the more likely he or she will be to make a suicide attempt.
2. People who don't feel pain when they self-injure are more likely than those who do to make a suicide attempt.
3. Kids who self-injure using multiple methods are more likely to make a suicide attempt than those who use just one method.

If any of these descriptions sound like your child, the earlier the intervention, the better the chance for a speedier recovery.

Freeing Your Child to Develop the Skills to Lead an Effective Life

Finally, deliberate self-harm undercuts a child's capacities to develop the ability to tolerate life's painful moments and to effectively problem-solve. We all need to know how to successfully handle the difficulties life throws our way. Deliberate self-harm is a short-term solution to long-term problems, like taking aspirin for recurring headaches. It produces almost immediate relief—and with the onset

> Self-injury is like taking aspirin for recurring headaches: the relief is almost immediate, but the pain is guaranteed to surface again.

of relief, the adolescent turns his attention away from the issues that precipitated the emotional dysregulation and takes comfort in feeling better.

Dan, 15 years old, and I were trying to get a better idea about what set
off his recent cutting. He and I had been working together for a little over 3
months.

"Yeah, so my girlfriend was just being a bitch," he said. "She doesn't like
the guys I hang out with. Well, I went over to her house with these friends
and she was just cold. I said, 'Screw this.' We just left. I was so mad at her I
didn't even say good-bye. I don't know, somebody had a bottle of Jack Daniels
and I just chugged about two-thirds of it in like one gulp."

"Man, that is a lot of alcohol to drink in a short period of time. What
were you thinking?" I asked.

"I wasn't thinking at all. Anyway, after I got home my parents smelled
the alcohol and busted me. They said we would have to talk about it in the
morning. I knew they were really mad. When I woke up, I felt horrible. They
came into my room and tried to talk about what happened. They really put
me in a lousy mood. I called my girlfriend to see if she might cheer me up, but
she just gave me grief about the night before. I was really mad. I was so mad I
couldn't even think straight," he said.

"And maybe a little sad and guilty?" I wondered.

"Yeah, I guess so. Anyway, after I hung up I went into the bathroom to
look for a razor. After I cut myself I felt a bit better, but then I began to think
of what a loser I am."

As you can see in Dan's story, when kids resort to the short-term strategy
of deliberate self-harm to manage emotional dysregulation, they are keeping
themselves from learning how to solve interpersonal problems and remaining
vulnerable to impulsive behavior and all the difficult consequences that follow. They have trouble thinking clearly. Furthermore, they begin to con-
solidate a view of themselves
as people who are defective,
weak, and worthless. Often at
this point the adolescents are
struggling more with their internal judgments about having
given in to self-injury than
with the patterns that bring

> *Among the many harmful repercussions
> of self-injury, a less obvious one is that
> it keeps children from developing the
> problem-solving skills they will need all
> their lives in relationships.*

on the emotional turmoil. Of course, without a clear understanding of these
patterns there can be no new learning of how to manage these potentially
painful situations. Consequently these kids become chained to their repetitive self-injury and stuck in misery.

Black-and-White Thinking

You have probably also noticed how often your child is prone to black-and-white thinking. From your child's perspective, the world seems to be neatly divided between what she can do and what she absolutely can't, between what is good and what is not, between what is fair and what is unfair. All the different shades and nuances that are part of living for you are unavailable to her. While all-or-nothing thinking is a hallmark of adolescents, it is a more prominent feature in kids who self-injure, and is especially dominant when they are emotionally dysregulated.

How does this come about? In all likelihood black-and-white thinking, or what psychologists call "dichotomous thinking," results from an interaction between high emotional reactivity and an invalidating environment. As I mentioned earlier, when we get emotionally revved up, our thinking becomes rigid and constricted. We see things in terms of absolutes: "I will never get better" or "I can't make friends" or "I am stupid." Our emotions drive our thinking to make rigid categories for our experiences.

One consequence of an invalidating environment is that kids feel that life's problems should be easy to solve. The take-home message for them is that most other people don't seem to be bothered by what trips them up, and if they were only better, stronger, or smarter, they would sail through life. Consequently, they are prone to oversimplifying life's complex problems. This effort at simplifying things requires them to disregard complexities.

As you can see, self-injury is a behavior that needs to be addressed quickly and effectively. Time is of the essence. Until recently there hasn't been a treatment that has been shown to be effective in helping these kids turn away from deliberate self-harm in a relatively short period of time. But dialectical behavior therapy has become the gold standard for helping these kids. In the next chapter I'll introduce you to this treatment.

4

DBT

THE RIGHT THERAPY FOR YOUR TEEN

As the parent of a child who self-injures, there's nothing you want more than to see the behavior stop. In Chapter 1 I talked about how searching for the hidden meaning behind self-harm doesn't tackle the problem directly. Consequently, forms of treatment that focus on uncovering such meaning can take a very long time to produce change. In this chapter I'll describe dialectical behavior therapy (DBT), the best treatment to help your child find ways other than self-injury to deal with his or her emotional vulnerability. DBT is more successful than other forms of psychotherapy or medication, but, as I'll discuss, some of these alternatives make for excellent supplementary treatment. Finally, I'll give you some pointers on finding a good therapist and determining whether your teen needs more sustained help than outpatient therapy can offer.

HOW DBT ADDRESSES WHAT YOUR TEEN DOES AND THINKS

DBT—a form of cognitive-behavioral treatment that was developed and tested in the late 1980s and early 1990s by Marsha Linehan and her colleagues at the University of Washington—was initially used to help suicidal women, but over time has been applied to a wide variety of psychological troubles. The cognitive part of cognitive-behavioral therapy helps people change by examining and challenging their prior unhelpful, unrealistic beliefs about themselves and their world (cognitive distortions).

The behavioral part helps people change by teaching and reinforcing new and effective behaviors. The behavioral component is in all likelihood a more powerful agent of change than the cognitive piece. After all, the challenge is to get your teenager to stop doing something that, while it serves a particular purpose, is clearly harming her terribly. A behavior is reinforced by anything that increases the likelihood that it will occur again. There are two types of reinforcement, both of which you may remember from the days your child was a toddler. Things that *positively* reinforce behavior—for example, praising a child after he thanks you for giving him a ride to his friend's house—may increase the likelihood of the desired behavior happening again. (In addition, that "thank you" may make it more likely that you'll be willing to give him the ride the next time, so he's reinforcing you too.)

Negative reinforcement occurs when something aversive is applied and then removed after a behavior has occurred, "aversive" being defined by the person's emotional response. For example, sending a child to her room for a timeout may be aversive for one kid, but for another it may be a chance to rest, play video games, or talk on the phone. Consider the child who must stay in the classroom during recess (the aversive condition) until he apologizes for his rude behavior to the teacher. Once he does, he's allowed to join his class at recess. So the teacher has reinforced apologizing.

In most cases the behavior of deliberate self-harm is under the control of negative reinforcement. Your child is feeling emotionally overwhelmed (the aversive condition), and self-harm brings immediate relief. Self-harm is now more likely to occur again because it resolved the child's painful emotional experience. One of the few examples of deliberate self-harm being under the control of positive reinforcement is for that very small group of children who hurt themselves to get attention.

As you know, teenagers who injure themselves also operate on a number of false or distorted beliefs that contribute to their urge to hurt themselves. This is where the cognitive part of cognitive-behavioral therapies comes in. A sad but common cognitive distortion held by kids who self-injure is that they are defective and weak.

"I did it again last night," Melanie told me. "I tried not to cut myself, but I just couldn't hold out. I don't think I have the willpower to stop."

"Your inability to refrain from cutting is not a function of willpower," I countered. "You have enormous capacity for willpower and self-discipline—just look at how focused you are on your schoolwork and sports. It's not willpower you lack, but the *skills* necessary to manage that high-powered emotional system of yours."

Melanie's distorted thinking is based on the faulty assumption that if she had more willpower, she wouldn't engage in deliberate self-harm. One aspect of a cognitive-behavioral therapist's job is to help the adolescent challenge this belief and to replace it with one that conforms to the facts about self-injury—specifically, that self-injury is most often due to lacking the skills to manage one's emotions.

> *DBT will teach adolescents new behaviors to finally help manage their emotions.*

In DBT the child is taught specific skills—new behaviors—that will help modulate and/or change painful emotions. While it is important to challenge these beliefs, the most powerful agent of change is helping the child learn a new behavior to replace the harmful one that serves the same function.

DBT: THE NATURAL ANTIDOTE

DBT directly targets the specific emotional and behavioral problems that plague the adolescent who deliberately self-injures. One of the key components of DBT is to teach these adolescents the relevant skills to handle their powerful emotional system. DBT is not a miracle treatment. It doesn't help everyone, but to date it's the best and fastest treatment there is. Here's why.

Restores Emotion to Its Proper Status

Emotional dysregulation, as you now know, is likely at the root of your child's self-injuring behavior. You'll also recall that when a person is emotionally dysregulated and in need of help, offering a solution to her problem before helping her see that her emotional state is real and important can be a recipe for disaster; it skips the critical step of validating her emotional experience. Without validation, these adolescents come to believe that their emotions are exaggerated or untrustworthy, robbing them of the important information their emotions are sending them. This leaves them not only unsure of what to do in a specific situation but with a pretty shaky sense of self overall.

Linehan noticed that offering her patients techniques for change without first accepting and validating their experience kept them stuck, unable to move forward in treatment. Her Eureka! moment came when she tried incorporating acceptance strategies and validation into the treatment. Lo and behold, her patients began to get better.

The following example illustrates the importance of validation. Notice how stuck we get as I start with problem solving before validation.

Chloe paged me because she felt so depressed and lethargic that she didn't feel able to get her laundry done for an upcoming weekend at a friend's house.

"I have no energy. I just want to get into bed," Chloe complained.

"I know you want to see your friend—you've really been looking forward to this trip for a long time. Maybe if we break the tasks into smaller pieces they won't seem so overwhelming," I suggested.

"I have no energy. I can't do anything," Chloe told me with some irritation.

"Has your goal of going on this trip changed?" I asked. "Because I know you could get your chores done if we came up with a plan."

"I don't think you understand. This is not easy," Chloe said with anger rising in her voice.

"I think maybe you're right. I haven't let you know that I do understand that the laundry and the rest of your chores feel just too hard to do when you feel this way."

"It feels impossible for me to do anything when I feel this way."

"You are really up against it. You really want to see your friend, and the things you need to do to make that happen feel like trying to swim with lead shoes on," I said.

"I do want to go, I'm just feeling like there's no way I can make it happen," she said. "It makes me feel hopeless."

"No wonder you're feeling up against it," I said. "Would you like some help problem solving?"

"Yeah. What do you think I should do?"

Moves between Acceptance and Change

In a DBT treatment we are always moving between accepting and validating things as they are and looking for solutions to bring about change. This constant moving back and forth led Linehan to the concept of dialectics—she put the "D" in DBT.

Dialectics is a complicated concept and one that often trips up therapists as well as parents, so I won't get into a long explanation of what the word means. Suffice it to say that in DBT it frees parents and teens, or therapists and teens, from the polarized points of view that stand in the way of change. When our positions are polarized, each side has a tendency to dig their heels in and cling tightly to their view of the truth. The discussion now is characterized by the issues being black or white, and all the colorful shades in the middle are lost. When we are thinking dialectically, we come to understand that truth is neither absolute nor relative (except in the case of things like gravity or the temperature at which water boils at sea level vs. in the mountains).

The idea is that in most interpersonal encounters, no one individual holds the whole truth; rather, each has a piece of it. I've already spoken about this in relation to learning to let go of your own dearly held position in order to work with others toward a solution. In DBT, we take this notion a step further, learning to build a more complete understanding that goes beyond the simple sum of our combined truths. In fact, one helpful device for moving into dialectical thinking is to begin looking for what's left out of each person's position. (Can you think of anything more at odds with the black-and-white thinking that is often a hallmark of kids who self-injure?)

Two versions of a dialogue between Jenna and a therapist portray a typical impasse. The therapy can't move forward until the patient and the therapist find a way to get unstuck.

JENNA: BREAKING THROUGH THE IMPASSE

"I can't do it! I can't just tolerate that awful feeling. Do you think I cut myself for no reason? You make it all sound so easy. You never really get it, do you?" Jenna said as she began to cry.

"I don't make it sound so easy. I think *you* misunderstand me. I'm only trying to help you reach your goals."

There isn't a shred of dialectical thinking going on here. Jenna and her therapist are at the opposite ends of the spectrum. They need to search for *what is left out* or not being articulated in each other's points of view. Here's an alternate scenario.

"I can't do it! I can't just tolerate that awful feeling. Do you think I cut myself for no reason? You make it all sound so easy. You never really get it, do you?" Jenna said as she began to cry.

"You know, I think you're right. When I talk about using skills, I can give the impression that it's simple. What I want you to know is that *simple* is not the same as *easy*. This is really hard work. It makes sense to me that you would feel misunderstood. We have to work together to help you stop cutting."

"Yeah, I really feel like no one gets how hard this is. I feel like you can't possibly understand what it's like to be me."

"I guess I need to pay more attention to that. I do see how hard you're trying, and I want to keep encouraging you."

"That would help. I know sometimes I back myself into a corner," Jenna replied. "You know, it isn't that I can't do this—only that I'm not very good at it yet. I sometimes get angry at you, but mostly I'm just frustrated with myself."

Here Jenna and her therapist are both looking for what was left out of the discussion in the first example. The therapist validates Jenna's experience and moves between acceptance and change so that they can work more collaboratively toward progress.

As a parent you most likely have had the experience of finding yourself and your partner on opposite sides of an issue. Let's say your teenager comes home 2 hours past her curfew, but she called 10 minutes before curfew to say that she'd be home in an hour or so. This was something new; often she'd be late and not call. Your partner's view is that at least she called—he wants to support that improvement by not giving your daughter a consequence. You think she should be given a consequence because she was late.

You both feel strongly about the correctness of your positions, and neither of you is budging. Before long things heat up. You tell your partner that he's too lenient. He tells you that you're being too hard on the kid. But if you could both step back, you'd be able to see that each of your positions includes some truth and excludes some truth. Once you realize that each of you holds a legitimate piece of the truth, you'll find a way both to acknowledge your daughter's new be-

> *To engage in the dialectical thinking at the heart of DBT, we need to see that each person's position has some truth to it. The dialogue can then be a series of building blocks that go beyond any one individual's point of view.*

havior and to give a consequence for her being late: "We're glad that you called us to let us know you were safe and what time to expect you. That's the first time you've done that, and we noticed it and appreciated it. But we're still concerned that you came home 2 hours after your curfew, so you're grounded next Friday."

JAMIE: THE TRUTH, THE DIALECTICAL TRUTH, AND NOTHING BUT THE DIALECTICAL TRUTH

Why is dialectical thinking superior to other types of reasoning? If we held truth to be *absolute*, we would conclude that deliberate self-harm is either good or bad. A parent would take one position and the child who self-injures would take its opposite. With no common ground, the situation would generate a great deal of noise and smoke but very little light.

Seeing truth as *relative* would have the parents taking a position like this one: "Self-injury is not something we would do, but it's your body to manage as you see fit. We can only hope that in time you'll stop." The adolescent's position would go something like this: "I know you don't like what I do, but you respect my decisions to manage my body as I choose, since my behavior is not hurting anybody else." This position is very democratic—but it's not going to solve anything.

If we were to think *dialectically* about self-injury, however, the dialogue would be a series of building blocks that would go beyond any one person's point of view. It's exemplified by Jamie and her father, who came to see me about her cutting. Their conversation quickly got off track.

"You just have to stop hurting yourself, Jamie. There's no way around this. It's just not right!" said Jamie's dad with some tension in his voice.

"You can't stop me, and it's my body, anyway," Jamie replied curtly.

"Jamie, can you tell your dad about how your cutting helps you?" I interjected.

"I could, but I don't think he cares," she responded.

"Give me a try," her dad said, somewhat incredulously. "I'm curious about how it could possibly be helpful to you."

"Okay, but you have to listen."

Her dad nodded.

"I cut myself when I can't stand how overwhelmed I feel, and it calms me down. I know that sounds crazy, but it's true. I hate myself for doing it. I hate myself even more when you get angry at me about it," Jamie said, suddenly in tears.

"I'm not angry with you," her father said sympathetically. "I'm really more frightened for you. I want so badly for you to stop hurting yourself. I know I push you. I'm frustrated because nothing has worked and it's been going on for a long time. You've ignored me when I've tried to help."

"I haven't ignored you, Dad. You seem to think it's all about willpower, and it's not. Trust me, I don't really want to do it, and I've tried hard to stop, but right now I just can't. You have no idea how awful I feel right before I cut myself."

"It's hard for me to believe that hurting yourself really makes you feel better, but if it does, I guess I can understand why you keep doing it. I never knew that. I guess I thought you did it mostly to spite me. We have to help you find another solution for those times when you get overwhelmed," Jamie's dad said as he reached for her hand.

Notice in this conversation how each person adds a little more information that opens the possibilities for a new and expanded view of the problem—and real hope for a resolution. Jamie's dad gains an appreciation for the way his daughter's self-injury helps her and learns that Jamie really wants things to be different. Jamie learns that her father is willing to help her in the process of finding a solution to her emotional dysregulation while trying to be less judgmental. Thinking dialectically can open the door for real understanding and help parents and kids join together to find the path to close and effective relationships.

Heads Off Guilt and Self-Blame

In DBT your teen and you will be oriented to what is called the "biosocial theory" of self-injury. You've already been introduced to this theory in Chapter 2, without the ten-dollar name; it simply means that kids are prone to the kind of emotional upheaval that can lead to self-injury as a result of both biology and environment. Understanding this origin of your teen's problems helps both of you understand what went wrong without feeling like either of you has to take the blame. Your child is not "weak" or "defective" but simply endowed with a Ferrari of an emotional engine—a characteristic, incidentally, that has its plus sides too as it can, for example, imbue your teen with the passionate drive to pursue dreams and right injustices as an adult. The biosocial theory should also reassure you that your child is not having problems with emotional regulation because you are a bad parent.

The biosocial theory is just as important a foundation to DBT as dialectics because it not only explains what has gone wrong but, even more important, provides a kind of road map about how to get back on track. Your child needs to learn the skills necessary to manage her high-powered emotional system, and you need to find ways to help your teen view her emotions as real and significant. As you become more familiar with DBT, you'll probably feel a diminished sense of guilt as you come to see yourself and your child's' difficulties from a more compassionate perspective. Likewise, your teenager will understand that her troubles are not a function of some inherent character flaw or deficiency, but the understandable outcome of emotional dysregulation.

Mr. and Mrs. Roberts, two computer engineers, and their daughter, Regina, a lovely 15-year-old girl who was heavily into the arts, came to see me for a consultation. Regina had been self-injuring for the last year, and nothing her parents tried seemed to help. Her parents described her as being "overly emotional" and not able to think clearly. Regina's parents were confused and worried.

"We are very rational people and Regina can be just a bundle of emotions. When she gets like that, we just can't reason with her. It makes us think that we're not good parents," Mr. Roberts told me.

"It has nothing to do with you," Regina said. "You just don't understand! I can't help it if you guys don't have feelings. My parents are robots," she told me.

"We have feelings," Mrs. Roberts said. "We just don't let them get in the way of being rational."

"Are you telling me that I'm not rational?" Regina asked, getting ready for battle.

> *As he or she undergoes DBT, your teenager will understand that his or her self-injury is not the result of a character flaw but of emotional dysregulation—and that he or she can gain the skills to stop it.*

"I think it may be that there are some real differences in the way each of you experiences emotions. These differences may be part of the problem you all are having understanding each other. Understanding these differences can be an important first step in solving the problem," I suggested.

Directly Attacks Emotional Dysregulation from Multiple Angles

As I discussed in earlier chapters, emotional dysregulation affects all aspects of a child's life: managing cognitive processes, working toward goals, and developing a sense of identity. As your teenager becomes emotionally "fluent" over time, he will have enough practice in skillfully managing his emotions—either through change strategies, like "opposite action to current emotion" from the emotion regulation skills module or by learning how to tolerate them using the "crisis survival strategies" from the distress tolerance module—that he will not have to resort to deliberate self-harm.

I will introduce you to the skills that make all this possible a little later in the chapter. For now my point is that DBT directly targets emotional dysregulation in multiple ways by giving the teen a number of different skills that serve as direct replacements for self-injury.

Helps Teens Learn Who They Are and What's Right for Them

The development of a cohesive sense of identity is one of the core tasks of adolescence. Our sense of identity is a complicated set of interrelated strands that help give us that feeling of who we are, no matter what situation we find ourselves in. It has to be flexible enough so that the person we are when we are at home with our family can shift into the person we are at work. In addition, our sense of identity includes our ethical standards, values, and personal ambitions.

Developing a sense of identity is a complex process in which the child tries on various personas, tossing those that don't fit. If you're the parents of a child in early to middle adolescence, you know that this age is characterized by remarkably rapid changes in clothing styles, speech patterns, and interests. These kinds of behaviors help adolescents begin to define themselves. In order for this process to occur, they must be able to focus their attention on how they think and feel about themselves in relation to an array of interpersonal, ethical, and moral issues. This process of ongoing self-reflection requires adolescents to integrate clear thinking and emotional experience. They need to be able to modulate their emotions, to be mindful (more about this shortly) of their thoughts and feelings, and to validate the wisdom in their conclusions.

Clearly, an emotionally dysregulated adolescent is going to have a hard time with these tasks. She will not come easily to the statement "This is who I am, and this is what's right for me." Being unable to self-validate, she'll struggle to find a stable platform from which to declare her selfhood. Furthermore, this process occurs best when kids are not continually disrupted by extreme moments of emotional dysregulation—that is, finding oneself calls for quiet, reflective time.

The DBT therapist actively validates the child's growing sense of herself while working on helping her figure out her own set of values and teaching the skills she will need for self-validation.

Helps Teens Pay the Right Amount of Attention

When we are emotionally overwhelmed, our thinking either constricts and we become focused on too narrow a view, or our thinking becomes diffuse and we can't see the forest for the trees. As you've undoubtedly seen in your teenager, this loss of attentional control leads to poor decision making and is the fertile ground for the distorted thinking that often plagues these children. The DBT therapist helps the teen identify distorted thinking that results from a view that is either too concentrated or too scattered. Then the therapist teaches skills to keeping the view at just the right perspective.

Helps Teens Control Their Impulses

The terrible feeling of being emotionally overwhelmed often drives kids who self-injure to rush into impulsive and other risky, ineffective behaviors geared toward bringing short-term relief. It's not uncommon for them to take action without knowing what propelled them. In individual DBT, adolescent and therapist look step-by-step at what led to a behavior, the behavior itself, and its long- and short-term consequences. This step-by-step process is called a "behavior chain analysis"; each link in the chain represents a thought or a behavior that led to whatever problematic event is being investigated.

Many of the skills your teen will be taught in DBT wind up helping with impulse control too.

Like the cops in the old TV series *Dragnet*, the DBT therapist teaches patients to focus on "Just the facts, ma'am," rather than jumping to conclusions. Many of the skills youths learn in DBT—from mindfulness to emotion-regulation skills to interpersonal skills—help with impulse control too.

GAINING THE SKILLS TO SUCCEED

An important underlying assumption in DBT is that these teens' difficulties arise because they lack the skills to manage their powerful emotions. This skills deficit leads to behavioral problems, poor thinking and poor judgment, and an insecure sense of self. What can they do? Reckless sexual behavior, disordered eating, and, of course, deliberate self-harm can all calm down the adolescent who feels emotionally overwhelmed. Living life in an emotional whirlwind often makes interpersonal relationships difficult. And with their poor judgment and general sense of identity confusion, these kids are often at a distinct disadvantage when it comes to negotiating the normal tasks involved in becoming a competent adult.

DBT directly addresses these skills deficits, both in individual therapy and in skills-training groups. In individual treatment the DBT therapist and the adolescent review recent events and work at figuring out what would have been a more skillful approach to the situation. Together they may practice the new skill through role playing or the therapist may assign "homework." In skills-training groups the child is introduced to the four skills modules that are essential to DBT: mindfulness, interpersonal effectiveness, emotion regulation, and distress tolerance. Here I can only briefly describe what takes many sessions and hours of outside practice time for my adolescent patients.

Mindfulness

If there is one skill at the heart of DBT, it's mindfulness. *Mindfulness* is the capacity to focus one's attention *and* to have a broad enough perspective to take in new information. It's what we need in order to accurately identify and label our emotions. It's the capacity to stay present in our lives, doing what our circumstances require and accepting things as they are. Without mindfulness, the other necessary DBT skills can't be accessed.

We can do anything mindfully. For example, as a mindfulness practice I often suggest that teens pick an activity and just stay focused and present on what they are doing, whether it's walking, eating, or listening to music. In the language of DBT, I'm asking them to fully participate and to do this one thing mindfully. I ask them to notice when their mind wanders off the task, which it certainly will—that's how minds work—and to gently bring themselves back to the task at hand.

This ability is significantly compromised when we are swept away by our emotions. When these teens are emotionally revved up, it's extremely difficult for them to work at skillfully analyzing and planning what to do next. They often seem to be flailing from one idea to another, without the capacity to slow down and evaluate the most effective course of action. But mindfulness works at undercutting many of the problems associated with emotional dysregulation. As these kids practice it, they learn to stay focused on just what is, without either being swept away by their emotions or judging them as negative. Mindfulness practice helps kids know how to observe and describe their thoughts and emotions in a nonjudgmental way. As they become more proficient at this, they'll be much more competent at modulating and managing powerful emotions, and their thinking will stay on track.

> *Mindfulness—the ability to focus one's attention while having a broad enough perspective to take in new information—can be practiced while walking, eating, or listening to music. It can't take place when we are swept away by our emotions.*

Interpersonal Effectiveness

Teens who self-harm often have difficulty in interpersonal relationships. They may work hard at fitting in, but never really believe that they do. They're often very sensitive to perceived rejections, and so they guard against rejection and the accompanying sense of abandonment by holding on too tightly in relationships. Not surprisingly, this backfires and their friends often find them "clingy." Some children are daunted by the thought of making friends because they just don't have the skills to go about it. Sadly, the result is often that they're left out socially, or at best only marginally included in the adolescent community.

Helping them learn interpersonal effectiveness skills allows them to figure out what they're shooting for in an interpersonal situation. The first question they are asked to mindfully consider is, What is your priority for this interaction? Follow-up questions include: Are you asking for something? Trying to repair a relationship? Setting a limit that will help you hold on to your self-respect? And how do you want to feel about yourself after this interaction? Once those key questions are answered, the adolescent is taught to use interpersonal skills, practices them in therapy, and then applies them in real-life situations. Thus armed, these kids are able, often for the first time, to have successful friendships without the emotional tension they've been accustomed to.

Brandon, age 16, was telling me about his most recent argument with his mother. In the past he and his mom would frequently argue and not find any closure. He wouldn't apologize and she would just stay disappointed and resentful. The resulting tension between them could last for days and was often a contributing factor to his self-injury.

> *DBT teaches your child to practice interpersonal skills in therapy and in the real world. With increasing abilities, emotional tension in relationships begins to melt away.*

"I had a big fight with my mom on Saturday but this time it was different," Brandon told me. "Instead of walking away I used my new skills and tried to understand my mom's point of view, and I made an apology. It really worked!"

Emotion Regulation

As I've discussed at length, these kids don't have the skills to modulate their emotional distress. In DBT, they learn specific techniques that help them turn down the temperature on the emotional upheaval and increase the possibility for positive emotional experiences.

The emotion regulation module essentially targets dysregulation from three directions. First, kids are taught the value that emotions play in our lives as sources of communication, as aspects of self-validation, and as precursors to action.

> *Your child will learn specific techniques to help "turn down the temperature" on emotional upheaval.*

Second, they learn about all the ways we can become vulnerable to negative emotions and how managing our lives better can help us avoid being overwhelmed by them. Third, they learn some specific skills that can help change the way they are feeling. I demonstrate some of these techniques in the next chapter.

Distress Tolerance

We all know that there are some problems in life that can't be solved. They can be as mundane as being stuck in traffic or as heartbreaking as the death of someone dear to us. Some events in life are going to be painful no matter what, and we need a skill to help us through these tough times. Kids who en-gage in deliberate self-harm at such moments have a way of making the situa-tion worse, often through some kind of impulsive behavior or by doing some-thing that is interpersonally ineffective. The DBT skill set that helps us gets through these moments are the distress tolerance skills, which fall into two categories.

First are the skills we need to accept our current situation. Accepting things as they are does not mean that you're giving in or that you like the sit-uation. It only means you're acknowledging that things are happening the way they are at that moment and not fighting them. This set of skills is labeled the "basic principles of accepting reality." The second category com-prises the "crisis survival strate-gies," which are aimed at help-ing us get through the moment. They're not geared toward prob-lem solving; they just provide skills to temporarily diminish or distract us from our pain. Crisis survival strategies include doing

> The two parts of distress tolerance are accepting the situation and learning crisis survival strategies to get through the moment by diminishing our pain or distracting us from it.

things that are self-soothing, like taking a bubble bath, or distracting, like getting totally involved in knitting a sweater. I think the distress tolerance skills are one of the most important skill sets for parents to learn too as they go through worrisome times with kids who self-injure.

DBT: NOT "TREATMENT AS USUAL"

The following excerpt is from the last family meeting I had with Vicki and her parents.

Vicki, age 15, and I had worked together in DBT for a little over a year. We met once a week for individual therapy. She was also in a weekly skills group. Her folks attended a skills group for parents during the first 6 months of the treatment. Vicki came to therapy to help her stop cutting and to reduce her emotional outbursts. Her outbursts generally occurred when someone in her life disappointed her.

"Well, here we are, just about a year after we started. So what has changed for each of you and as a family?" I asked.

"Really, a lot has changed," Vicki's dad began. "I think I am much better at not jumping to problem solving with Vicki and my wife. It really helps things from becoming arguments."

"You have gotten better at that, Dad. Like on Sunday when I couldn't get my math homework and was starting to lose it. You didn't tell me I was being irrational, that all I needed to do was to focus better. You just validated how hard it was for me and asked if there was anything you could do to help. Then I didn't feel like such a jerk for having a hard time understanding my homework."

Vicki's mom spoke up. "He is better at validating, and I think we are both better at trying to think dialectically."

"Give me an example," I said.

"Well," she said, "when we disagree on things, we don't just go around and around trying to prove we're right. We understand that Vicki still gets upset and does things that we don't approve of. In the past I would be the understanding one and her dad would set the limit. Now we work hard at understanding each other's point of view—we get that we're both right."

"So this is great progress. Anything else?" I ask.

"I think I can speak for my wife here: we are just better at managing our worries. Sometimes when Vicki is getting worked up, we just remind ourselves to radically accept that this is her experience, and we can't talk her out of it or change it in the moment. We let her work it out herself, but stay close by. Those distress tolerance skills have helped us keep our anxiety from making the situation worse," Vicki's dad replied. "But enough about us. We are really proud of what Vicki has accomplished."

"I want to hear what she has to say."

"It's been 9 months and 17 days since I last cut myself," Vicki said with a clear sense of pride in her voice. "I never thought I'd be able to do that. I mean, I still get urges, but I feel like I know how to handle them now. I think the biggest thing for me is that I feel more in charge of my emotions. They can get pretty strong at times, like when I have a fight with my boyfriend. But if I use my mindfulness skills to observe and describe what is happening inside of me, then I can usually figure out what I should do next."

"Vicki, that is just tremendous. I can remember when you didn't have a clue about what you were feeling," I said. "Anything else?"

"Well," she said, "I think my parents would agree, we all get along much better these days. You would probably say we are more interpersonally effective," she said with a smile on her face.

The first studies that demonstrated DBT's effectiveness were published in the early 1990s. The treatment protocol called for a year of individual psychotherapy and a year of skills training in a group. These studies examined DBT in comparison to a "treatment as usual" group who underwent longer term "talk therapy" with private therapists and in mental health centers. The researchers found, among other things, that compared to people who received treatment as usual, those undergoing DBT showed a significantly lower rate of deliberate self-harm, lower rates of suicide attempts, and fewer days spent as inpatients in psychiatric hospitals.

Although it was not designed specifically to treat adolescents, toward the mid-1990s Alec Miller, Jill Rathus, and Marsha Linehan developed an adapted version of DBT for the adolescent who was suicidal, engaged in deliberate self-harm, or exhibited various other forms of high-risk behavior. The adolescent would be seen once a week in individual DBT, and he or she participated in a weekly multifamily skills group with a parent or guardian.

> *Adolescents in DBT who had been self-harming injured themselves less often, attempted suicide less often, and dropped out of therapy less often compared with those in more conventional therapy.*

The treatment was shortened from the standard of 1 year to just 12 weeks, and the skills group always included the adolescent's parent or guardian.

In 1998 my colleagues and I started an intensive outpatient program in our Cambridge, Massachusetts, offices for adolescents for whom DBT appeared to be the best treatment. Many of them were engaged in self-harm and/or struggling with suicidal ideas, depression, and eating disorders. The program works the same way today. The adolescents meet as a group 5 days a week for 4 hours a day, during which time they're taught the full curriculum of DBT skills.

> *Parents are actively involved in both their child's individual and group therapies.*

They also meet individually with a DBT therapist once or twice a week. Parents are actively involved in the program through weekly contact with the child's therapist and in their attendance in a DBT skills group.

The children who meet with success in our program are not "cured" in a few short weeks. They do, however, make significant progress. See Appendix A for a detailed assessment of the outcomes for 42 adolescents treated during 2005–2006. In summary, there was a significant decrease in adolescents' experience of depression, anxiety, anger, and other forms of psychological distress, back to within normal range. In addition, symptoms of borderline personality disorder and self-injurious thoughts and behaviors showed significant improvement, as did the development of emotion regulation skills and functioning at home and in social situations.

In my experience DBT can help kids dramatically reduce self-harming behavior in 3 to 6 months, as well as reduce overall feelings of psychological

> *DBT can help kids dramatically reduce self-harming behavior in 3 to 6 months. They also experience reduced overall psychological distress and depression and improve their ability to regulate their emotions and functioning in all domains of their lives.*

distress and depression. Often they continue meeting in weekly individual and skills-group sessions for another 6 months to a year. The additional treatment helps them hold on to the gains they have made and sustain a more normalized teenage life for themselves.

Over the years there have certainly been kids who didn't benefit from DBT, either because I wasn't skilled enough to help them or because they had life experiences that stacked the deck too solidly against them. For the most part, however, the hundreds of kids I have seen in individual therapy or who have gone through our program who learned the DBT skills, practiced them in daily life, and worked at understanding the triggers for their self-injury showed positive results. One of the best parts of my professional life is that patients sometimes return after

> *The "guarantee" I give my patients is that if they learn these new skills, practice them outside the office, and work to understand the triggers for their self-injury, they will see positive results.*

months or years to tell me how they're doing. Over the last 10 years most of them have stopped self-injuring—and in a shorter period of time than with any other treatment.

WHAT ABOUT OTHER TYPES OF PSYCHOTHERAPY?

Very few studies have examined the effectiveness of other therapies on treating self-injury. You may encounter therapists who use psychodynamic therapies (treatments that focus on how the teen's past is being re-enacted in the present and use this insight to bring about change), CBT, and integrative therapies (a mixture of different treatment approaches). To ascertain whether a particular approach may be useful for your teen, I suggest you ask each potential therapist "Is the therapy going to directly target self-harm, or is the treatment going to resolve self-injurious behavior by a more indirect route by helping the child resolve the problems that lead to the behavior?"

HOW TO FIND A DBT THERAPIST

The good news is that DBT has been adapted to bring swift and lasting help to teens who self-harm. The not-so-good news is that because it's a relatively new treatment, finding a trained therapist isn't always easy. Each year, though, more and more therapists are learning DBT. One way to find a therapist is to consult the online list, arranged by location, at *www.behavioraltech.org*. Behavioral Tech is the national organization that provides training to clinicians and serves as a resource for consumers interested in DBT. While Behavioral Tech can't vouch for the *kind* of training these therapists have received, it's a good start to hunting one down in your community.

Another route is a hunt-and-peck approach, or networking. Start by asking your managed care providers if they know of DBT therapists. Sometimes the state association of psychologists and social workers can be a good resource. Also, call your local community mental health clinic and any local hospitals that have child psychiatry outpatient clinics.

Your sources for locating a DBT therapist include:

1. Consult the list, arranged by location, at *behavioraltech.org*.
2. Ask around, starting with your child's doctor.
3. Check out your state's association of psychologists and social workers.
4. Phone a local mental health clinic or local hospital and find out whether they have child psychiatry outpatient clinics.

When you do locate a potential DBT therapist, there are certain key questions you should ask. Has he or she attended the intensive training course offered by Behavioral Tech, the major teaching program for DBT? Or did the therapist learn the treatment in graduate school? Is he or she part of a consultation team of other DBT therapists? The consultation team is an essential aspect of DBT. Its role is to help the therapist stay on track with the DBT. Is there a mechanism for skills coaching apart from formal sessions? Finally, does the therapist work with adolescents? While it is very useful for a therapist to have attended intensive training, it shouldn't be a deal breaker. In such cases, however, questions 2 and 3 become much more critical in determining your decision.

> Is this the right therapist for my child?
>
> 1. Has the therapist undergone an intensive training course?
> 2. Will there be a whole consultation team?
> 3. Is there a clear mechanism for skills coaching outside the therapy hour?
> 4. Has the therapist worked extensively with adolescents?

Guidelines for Choosing the Right Therapist

Individual therapy in all likelihood is going to be the central treatment plan for your teen's recovery, so make sure both your teen and you feel comfortable with the therapist. You should feel that you can trust and collaborate with this person and that you'll get your questions answered before and during treatment. That said, having a good relationship with the therapist is not enough.

Theoretical Orientation

The therapist needs to have a theory to help guide the treatment. I always find it worrisome when I speak with colleagues who tell me they don't have a particular theoretical orientation, or that they "just do what works." Psychological theories aid therapists in putting their patients' behavior in understandable contexts that generate useful and relevant interventions. If you're talking to someone who's not a DBT therapist, ask the therapist which theoretical orientation guides his or her understanding of kids who self-injure. Make sure you understand as completely as you can how the theory plays out in the actual implementation of the therapy.

Degrees and Experience

In my experience academic degrees are less important than the following, in this order:

1. The therapist should have at least several years of experience working with people who self-injure and should be able to explain how the particular therapy is going to address the issue.
2. The therapist should be considered to have expertise in working with adolescents.
3. The therapist should be clear about the parents' role in the treat-

ment and about the limits and extent of therapist–patient confidentiality.

SUPPLEMENTARY THERAPIES

Sometimes the DBT therapist may recommend additional therapy to support the DBT treatment. Whatever therapy is recommended needs to be aimed at helping the child become more adept at managing his or her emotions. What follows is a brief discussion of the supplementary therapies your practitioner is most likely to suggest.

Family Therapy

Family therapy, one of the most commonly prescribed additional treatments, rests on the premise that factors within the family are contributing to an individual's troubles; if these can be identified and remedied, the family system can help resolve them. As useful as family therapy can be, however, it often calls forth powerful and challenging emotions. If you've ever participated in family therapy, you know what I mean. If you haven't, just imagine sitting in a session with your child and other family members and trying to have a discussion about the cutting and other sensitive family matters. Family therapy requires kids who self-injure to employ one of the abilities they most sorely lack: modulating their emotions.

Not surprisingly, this group of kids typically manages family treatment in three ways: (1) they become mostly mute and seemingly brain-dead, (2) they are willing to engage in discussions only about the most mundane topics, and/or (3) they become emotionally charged and head for the door at the speed of light.

If family therapy is recommended, here are a few suggestions that may help make it more workable. First, get a clear sense of what both the individual therapist and the prospective family therapist envision as the task of the treatment. A red flag should go up if you hear things like the sessions being an opportunity for family members to express their feelings or open up channels of communication—excellent ideas in principle, but open-ended discussions may be beyond what your child (or you) can manage at this moment. If it's impossible for you to approximate these kinds of discussions at home without psychological meltdown, you're not going to have much more success in the therapist's office. On the other

> *Be prepared: family therapy can be emotionally intense.*

hand, if the therapist outlines the task of the treatment as a highly structured opportunity to learn and practice the skills required for effective communication and emotional regulation, sign up on the spot.

Second, as the poet said, timing is all. Think about whether it makes sense to wait on family therapy until your kid has developed some emotion regulation skills. There is very little mileage in going to family therapy and engaging in an important but emotionally charged discussion that dysregulates your kid, who then goes home and cuts.

In lieu of family therapy, it may be more useful to become involved in something focused on guiding parents. Generally, mental health professionals who have been trained to work with children also learn the skills necessary to be helpful to parents. Such sessions can help you become more skillful in responding to your teen's distress, managing your own worries about the troubles, and working successfully with your adolescent's therapist.

Group Psychotherapy

In typical adolescent group psychotherapy, four to eight kids meet on a regular basis with one or two clinicians. Groups can be time-limited—lasting, for example, only 12 sessions—or can continue for as long as the group members feel they're useful. Some groups have a theme—such as what it means to be a boy in modern U.S. culture—or a specific purpose, like teaching social skills. Often, however, they are open-ended, and participants can raise whatever issues feel most relevant to them. For most kids group therapy is very helpful because they often accept feedback that comes from a peer more readily than if it comes from an adult. But receiving any feedback on their issues is bound to be an emotionally charged experience, and adolescent group feedback is no exception.

Groups that are highly structured, skill–based, and limited in emotional expression can be the most useful for adolescents who self-injure. These are exactly what the DBT skills groups strive to do. (Sometimes kids are referred to a DBT skills group by their non-DBT therapist. While this won't do any harm, these kids are not going to get the full benefit of the treatment if they're not in both individual DBT and the DBT skills group.)

Medication

Psychopharmacology—psychiatric medication—is frequently an element of outpatient treatment for kids who self-injure. Referrals to a psychopharmacologist will usually be made by the individual therapist. If you have questions about whether medications might be useful for your child, I encourage you to ask the therapist and arrange for a consultation. Get a clear understanding of the benefits and the side effects of any medications that are being recommended. The best way to do this is to have your child seen by a qualified child psychiatrist or by an adult psychiatrist who sees a large number of children in his or her practice. Don't be shy: if you aren't clear about side effects, keep asking questions until you're satisfied that you know what to look for and what to expect.

Currently there are no medications that directly target deliberate self-harm. But there are several that offer indirect treatment to diminish emotional distress, lift mood, decrease impulsivity, and level out the extreme mood swings that are characteristic of these adolescents. Though they are rarely enough on their own, medications can be a great support of the child's work with the DBT therapist.

> *No medication specifically targets self-injuring behavior. But many can help indirectly by decreasing the emotional distress, impulsivity, and mood swings that contribute to the problem.*

Unfortunately, many of the psychiatric medications that are prescribed for kids have not been subjected to rigorous clinical trials with children. We know they work with adults, but we really can't say what the long-term effects might be on children. But depression and other psychiatric conditions in children can be incapacitating. In clinical practice we believe that not using the medications when they're indicated may make the situation worse.

The following brief descriptions of the more commonly used medications are offered only as a guideline to help you formulate questions to ask the prescribing physician.

Antidepressants

There are several classes of antidepressants, but the one most commonly prescribed are the selective serotonin reuptake inhibitors, or SSRIs. This class includes drugs like Prozac, Paxil, and Zoloft. Some of the SSRIs are thought to have a beneficial effect on anxiety, and can be prescribed when both depression and anxiety are part of the clinical picture. It's thought that people who suffer from depression lack sufficient quantities of serotonin in the brain, and the SSRIs remedy that by keeping more serotonin available for the brain to use. These medications usually don't begin to work for 4 to 6 weeks, so don't expect immediate results.

The SSRIs can be a very effective tool in the treatment of depression and, with the exception of two very important side effects that I will describe shortly, they are relatively benign. It is of the utmost importance, however, that you and the team with which you are working parse out what is true depression from the severe garden-variety unhappiness that may be enveloping your teen.

Side effects are an issue with any psychopharmacological regimen, and the SSRIs are no exception. Some side effects of the SSRIs are insomnia, stomach

> *Be sure the therapist is not mistaking your teen's profound unhappiness for depression. If he or she is not clinically depressed, antidepressants may not be of much help.*

distress, and minor muscle pain. These symptoms are generally mild and short-lived. Warning: children with undiagnosed bipolar disorder who take SSRIs face a more serious problem. This class of drug may induce manic episodes: racing thoughts, inability to sleep, increased agitation or irritability, grandiose ideas, and an abundance of energy that at first may seem a welcome contrast to the depressed mood, but soon leads to bigger problems. If your child seems overenergized after a couple of doses of an antidepressant, call the prescribing doctor.

A second serious side effect of the SSRIs, one that's been much in the news but that remains somewhat controversial, is that they may increase suicidal thinking. These medications even carry a "black box warning" (a cautionary note required by the FDA enclosed in a black box on the package insert). While all classes of antidepressant have been known to be somewhat energizing and sometimes this newfound energy is directed toward self-destructive thinking, the controversy surrounds some evidence that the SSRIs may bring this about in children more often than in adults. The side effect appears to be present in 2 to 4% of the children who are prescribed this class of medication. If you even suspect that your child is experiencing suicidal ideas after starting an antidepressant, let your doctor know immediately.

Mood Stabilizers

The mood stabilizers do just what their name implies: they stabilize the patient's moods by ironing out the extreme fluctuations to which these kids are often prone.

"It's like he's Dr. Jekyll and Mr. Hyde," Brian's mother told me. "One minute all is good in the world, and in the next he's down on himself and everything and everybody else."

There are essentially three classes of medications used as mood stabilizers.

The one that's been around the longest is lithium. Doctors who were treating gout patients with lithium first noted its mood-stabilizing effect 200 years ago, but the drug wasn't approved for the treatment of mood disorders until the late 1970s. Patients taking lithium need to have periodic bloodwork done to assess that the lithium level is not too high, which can be toxic to the body. In addition, they often experience considerable weight gain (a side effect that is unfortunately present in many of the medications used to stabilize kids' moods).

The second class of mood stabilizers are anticonvulsant medications such as Depakote, Lamictal, and Topamax; although it is not completely clear why these medications succeed in stabilizing moods, it is clear that they often do. Some require that blood levels be drawn periodically and some don't. They have some propensity to cause weight gain, with the exception of Topamax, which can suppress appetite. A side effect of Topamax that kids sometimes experience is a kind of slowing down or sluggishness to their thinking.

The third kind of mood stabilizer is a low dose of antipsychotic medications, especially the class known as the atypicals. Medications in this group include Risperdal, Seroquel, and Zyprexa. In addition to their mood-stabilizing effect, these medications can be used to treat anxiety, sleep issues, and impulsivity. As with the other mood stabilizers, the atypicals can cause significant weight gain and have been linked to an increase in diabetes. And even at very low doses, they sometimes produce a kind of lethargy and a feeling of deadness in a child.

Anti-anxiety Medications

Sometimes a psychiatrist will prescribe a benzodiazepine to help a child manage her anxiety. Medications like Ativan, Xanax, and Klonopin are all examples of anti-anxiety medications. They usually do a very good job of diminishing the child's experience of anxiety, and are often reasonable short-term solutions to overwhelming anxiety.

Being overwhelmed with anxiety is a horrible feeling. And often what we're anxious about are situations in which there is little reason to worry or our worry is out of proportion to the situation. For example, being anxious about going to a party where you will only know a few people may be reasonable, but becoming so overwhelmed with worry that you can't leave the house is a problem. There's a good chance that if you're overwhelmed with worry and take a benzodiazepine, you'll feel better in 20 minutes and can probably make it to the party.

The next time a similar situation arises, however, you will have to medicate yourself again. My personal philosophy of treatment (and this is just one person's point of view) is that anxiety is part of life; it's important to develop the skills to manage it, and cognitive-behavioral therapy can help.

There's no doubt that anti-anxiety medications can be of tremendous help when acute anxiety strikes. But the down side is that they can be addictive, so they can't be used regularly in the long term. If your child is prescribed one of these medications, make sure a clear exit strategy has been set up, or that the medications are limited to times of dire need. Furthermore, these medications can have a disinhibiting effect—that is, they may cause some kids to become more impulsive, which can lead to increased incidences of self-harm. This side effect seems more likely to occur in families with a strong history of alcoholism.

> *These particular medications can be addictive and should not be used long-term. If your child needs to go on one of them, make sure there is a clear exit strategy.*

If your child's psychiatrist recommends medications and has answered all your questions, I suggest that you give them a try and see how your child tolerates the regimen. Then you and your child have to carefully weigh the benefits versus the drawbacks. For example, if your kid has a history of poor judgment that leads to dangerous behavior, then the benefits from the medications may outweigh their drawbacks. On the other hand, if your child is actively involved in school, sports, and friendships and his self-injury is limited to times of interpersonal conflict, then the drawbacks of the medications may outweigh their benefits.

When the DBT and possible medications aren't enough help for your child, it may be time to consider more intensive inpatient or outpatient treatment programs.

Here is a set of guidelines that will help you, in conjunction with your child's treatment team, decide whether a more intense intervention is called for:

1. Is your child in imminent danger of suicide or seriously reckless behavior that compromises his or her safety?
2. Is your child's behavior unmanageable in your home, putting other family members at physical or emotional risk?
3. Are you and other members of your kid's support network so burned out that you need some respite?

If the answer to one or more of these questions is "Yes," a more comprehensive and containing treatment environment may be required.

It can be upsetting to realize your child needs this level of intervention, but when it's called for, the right program can be of tremendous benefit. A full discussion of these programs can be found in Appendix B.

YOUR INSURANCE COVERAGE

"Last Saturday was a nightmare. Susie had been out with friends and returned early, way before her curfew. Right there and then, we knew something was wrong. She came in the house with barely a hello and went right upstairs to her bathroom. When my husband and I checked in on her, she had cut herself and was beginning to put every pill she could find in her mouth," Susie's mom told me.

"That must have been scary! Did you call 911?" I asked.

"We sure did, and in some crazy way that was when the nightmare really began. It was about 11:00 when Susie was rushed to the emergency room. Initially things went really well—they attended to her medical condition immediately and told us a psychiatrist would be down to see us. Once she was medically clear, though, we sat for hours waiting to be seen by a psychiatrist. The psychiatrist arrived around 3:15; she spent 20 minutes with Susie and told us she thought Susie should be admitted to a child psych ward and that she would begin that process. An hour and a half later, the psychiatrist returned to say that she had found a bed at one of the local hospitals and that Susie would be transported there immediately.

"That was early Sunday morning. On Monday Susie's social worker from the hospital called and asked some questions about Susie and our family. On Wednesday my husband and I were invited to the discharge meeting. We were told that Susie was stabilized and that the managed care worker wanted to step Susie down, as she no longer met criteria for inpatient care. Susie's team told us that this was standard these days and that the hospital team would work to put an outpatient program in place.

"My husband and I were flabbergasted! I told the team that I had checked my insurance benefits and I knew we had 60 days per calendar year of inpatient coverage. The social worker let me know that the benefits were managed and that Susie would have to be discharged. We weren't sure Susie would be safe at home."

Some of you may have "been there and done that and have the pictures on the fridge." When it comes to private health insurance, there are several important facts for you, as customer, to know.

Negotiating managed care can be extremely frustrating. It's sometimes

1. What are the specific benefits that your plan allows for mental health? Make sure you are clear on the inpatient benefits as well as benefits for day hospital, and outpatient visits.
2. Does your plan allow for out-of-network coverage, or are you limited to the providers on the plan's list? If you can go out of network, what is the cost to you?
3. Is there any way to flex your benefits? For example, sometimes an insurance plan will flex, or make a swap, for inpatient benefits for partial hospital days.
4. If your child is a high user of clinical services, some managed care outfits have intensive care managers, who can sometimes go beyond the strict benefits allowed in your policy.

easier to bear the frustration when you keep in mind that the people who work for the managed care company are in a tough spot trying to make sure that your child is getting what he or she needs while at the same time following their company's protocol for services. Your best bet is to work in a collaborative relationship, advocating for your child's needs while understanding that it's not the managed care person on the phone who's the problem but the insurance coverage. Your role as the customer of a particular health insurance may give you the best leverage.

The criteria for accessing public insurance (Medicaid and Medicare) and public programs vary by state. Some states have relatively comprehensive services for people who depend on public programs, while others fall woefully short. While it often takes some detective work, you should find out about all the clinical services available for children in your state. Then begin to advocate for what your child needs. Patience and perseverance are the key ingredients. Don't give up!

I hope these chapters have given you a clearer understanding of the nature and genesis of your child's problems, and of the good news about the relatively new therapy that can make a big difference fast. In the next part of the book, I'll show you how to apply all the strategies and skills of DBT to your own dealings with your child. This therapy will give you a whole new way of interacting, installing validation as a core ingredient. It will also reduce stress in the family overall, and possibly even between you and your parenting partner. I'll also share some ways you can reinforce the positive effects of the DBT at home and some advice about talking with the people in your child's world—other family members, friends, teachers—about your child's difficulties.

PART II

helping your teen in treatment and at home

5

making the most of DBT

In this chapter I want to bring you into my office and let you see what happens in a DBT psychotherapy. Parents are too often in the dark about the process of treatment and therefore not in a position to assess whether the therapy is appropriate for their child, or even whether it's working. Psychotherapy may be a mixture of art and science, but it's not some mysterious process that can't be explained. By the end of the chapter you will understand the different components of DBT and how each treats the specific problems that contribute to deliberate self-harm.

In addition, I want you to have a better understanding of the times when you might be involved in the therapy, as well as those times when you're going to have to stay on the sidelines and let the process unfold. All therapists think a little differently about parental involvement. Use this chapter as a guideline for discussing it with the therapist. When you know what to expect, you'll feel less anxious and you'll be much more effective at supporting your child's treatment.

Please keep in mind that the treatment may often feel like two steps forward and one step back. The best way to assess whether it's working is to think of it as a stock: Is the trend going in the right direction over time? In moments of high emotional turmoil it won't be easy to tell whether progress is being made. For this reason I suggest that you keep a weekly chart to monitor your child's progress. I will have more to say at the end of the chapter about how you can assess whether progress is being made and what you can do to support your child's therapy.

> *Assessing the treatment is like watching a stock. What matters is whether the trend is going in the right direction over time.*

HELPING TEENAGERS CHANGE:
A CRITICAL BALANCING ACT

Therapists who work with adolescents have to be able to relate to them without losing their adult perspective. To be effective, I need to hold multiple perspectives (i.e., think dialectically) and continuously move back and forth between direct, honest communication and genuine curiosity and interest. Adolescents are notoriously allergic to phoniness and pomposity, and they will quickly become disenchanted with a therapist who is stiff and rigid, regardless of how knowledgeable that therapist may be. I sometimes think that working with adolescents is like walking a tightrope over a large tank that is divided in two. If I move too close to trying to be the adolescent's buddy in the service of establishing the relationship, I render myself useless as a re-

> *Therapists need to listen to their adolescent patients as if their story were the headline of the day, all the while knowing that tomorrow's paper will have a new headline.*

source and fall into the side of the tank that's full of sharks. But if I come across as a know-it-all adult, the kid tunes me out and pushes me into the other tank, this one filled with piranhas. The key is to strike a balance between being seen as someone who has something to offer and someone who has something to learn. I am most effective with my adolescent patients when I listen to them as if their story were the headline of the day, knowing that tomorrow's paper will have a new headline. See Chapter 8 for ideas on how you can do the same.

WHO, WHAT, WHERE, AND WHEN—
THE NUTS AND BOLTS

As I've explained, the standard protocol for outpatient DBT is a weekly individual session that lasts from 50 minutes to an hour, plus a weekly skills group for an hour and a half. In addition, kids have access to their DBT therapist after hours in times of crisis. It's customary for the therapist to ask for a particular time commitment. In our clinic that commitment is 6 months, after which the involved parties come together to review progress.

In my opinion, with very few exceptions, parents need to be involved in their child's treatment. I strongly recommend that you find out at the start of therapy what form that will take. The parents' involvement can be meeting regularly with the child and the therapist on a regular schedule, or just meeting as needed. Some clinics have parents come to a multiple-family skills group, where several families come together to learn the DBT skills.

INGREDIENTS OF YOUR CHILD'S DBT

Biosocial theory: A powerful tool to help your child see the self-harm in a new way and let go of the misguided, destructive idea that he or she is weak or defective.

Commitment to therapy: Your child must make an explicit commitment to the requirements of the therapy before the therapist can proceed.

Consultation team: The therapist must be involved with a team he or she can consult as needed during the therapy.

Between-session skills coaching: Your child must have 24/7 phone access to the therapist to help implement skills when needed.

Diary card: Your child needs to keep a record of any engaging in the target behaviors.

Skills practice: Using the new DBT skills in real life.

In the first phase of therapy the therapist has several important goals. Many therapies fail because this foundation for the treatment has not been cemented. Please review the checklist carefully. If your child's therapist doesn't raise these issues, make sure you do. Most of the rest of this chapter will cover these five essential steps.

THE FIVE ESSENTIAL THERAPIST GOALS TO BEGIN DBT

1. Talk with the adolescent enough to get a clear idea about what they're going to work on, and get her to commit to the requirements of DBT treatment.
2. Give the child and her parents a clear idea of how her problems developed, using the biosocial theory (more about this later).
3. Figure out whether the patient and the therapist are a good match, and highlight the importance of keeping channels of communication open.
4. Have an open discussion with the adolescent and her parents about what will remain confidential and what won't.
5. Outline how the parents are going to be included in the therapy.

ESTABLISHING THE GOALS OF TREATMENT
AND GETTING A PRELIMINARY COMMITMENT

All psychotherapies are a collaborative endeavor. With DBT this is particularly important. The adolescent and the therapist have to be a team working toward common goals. Without an open and collaborative relationship, very little therapeutic work can be accomplished. It is, in part, the work of the therapist to help the adolescent see the need for change and get him or her to make a commitment to the therapy.

This is delicate work. The key is to validate the wisdom in the child's behavior while exposing its ineffectiveness. Often the first step in this process is to have a discussion with the adolescent about his or her short-term and long-term goals. The trick is to link the goals to the need for change. We know that DBT does not begin until the adolescent makes a commitment to it. We also know that this commit-

> *Assessing your adolescent's commitment to therapy will be an ongoing process. The therapist and the patient will revisit it many times over the course of the therapy.*

ment is going to wax and wane. Assessing the adolescent's commitment to therapy is an ongoing process that therapist and patient will revisit many times over the course of therapy.

Parents can support their child's commitment to treatment in a variety of ways, from helping to finance the treatment and providing transportation to actively praising the child for the time and effort she's putting into it. Ultimately the matter of commitment is between your child and the therapist. Some parents hold out consequences if the child refuses to participate. Some clinicians may find this acceptable, but I don't think patients can work to change if the sole reason they're in therapy is because their parents want them to be.

TIFFANY: MAKING A COMMITMENT

Tiffany was a 15-year-old sophomore who was referred when her school counselor learned that she had been burning herself. She and her parents came to the first session together. I could tell everybody was a bit anxious and tense. The following discussion occurred about 20 minutes into our meeting.

"Okay, so you have been burning yourself for about 2 years now as a way to manage those awful feelings that come when you think you're going to do poorly at school. Do I have that right?" I asked.

"Yes, that's the only time I do it, but sometimes it happens a lot," she explained. "Up until recently nobody knew, and everything was fine. You know, I'm not sure if I really want to stop."

"We had no idea she was doing this! We've tried to talk with her about it, but we don't get too far. All that happens is that we get into an argument," Tiffany's mom reported.

"Self-injury can be a very difficult topic for kids and parents to discuss," I said gently. "Hopefully by the end of today you will have a better idea about what the behavior is all about and how we are going to address it." Turning to Tiffany, I asked, "It really keeps you calm, does it?"

"Yeah. I think I just need to do it less, and then it won't be a problem. Especially if I keep it quiet."

"Oh come on, Tiffany!" her dad quickly interjected. "That is just crazy behavior."

"I certainly understand your worry and how strange Tiffany's behavior appears," I said. "In some ways it actually makes a lot of sense." I turned my attention back to Tiffany. "So, what do you want to do after high school?" I asked her.

"I want to go to college. I know what you're going to think of this, but I want to be a child psychologist. I think I might be good at it," she offered.

"That's terrific. We really need people who want to work with kids . . . but hold on a minute, what about the burning? Becoming a psychologist means going to college and then graduate school, and school seems to be a big-time stressor for you. Besides that, how would you feel if you were still engaged in burning when you were treating kids?" I asked. "Don't you think that might be a problem?"

"I wasn't really thinking that far ahead. I guess I kinda assumed I would be able to stop it by then. If I was still doing it, I could see how that might be a problem. I would feel kind of phony trying to help kids if I was still burning myself," Tiffany said. "But I'll stop it when I'm older."

"Actually, without treatment, self-injury often continues into adulthood. What do you think is going to change for you to make it possible to stop?" I asked.

"I don't know—maybe I'll just get better at dealing with stress."

"How do you think you can do that?" I wondered.

"Other people manage it without hurting themselves. I assume I can too," she replied.

"You're absolutely right." I said. "But I suspect you might need some help figuring out how to tolerate some really uncomfortable feelings. Are you interested?"

"Yes," she said. "I don't want this thing to get in the way of going to school and doing what I want to do."

"Great," I replied. "It's going to be hard work to change this kind of behavior, but together I know we can do it."

Getting Everyone on Board

Tiffany's story describes the first step in the process of assessing which behaviors are going to be targeted in therapy and beginning to make a commitment. I like to have parents attend the first session or two so I can meet them and give them a sense of the person who is going to be meeting with their child. I want everyone involved to get an idea about how I think about self-injury and how we are going to work at resolving it. Not every therapist or DBT therapist works this way, but I believe it is critical to get you into the room at the start. The next steps include determining what other behaviors need targeting and getting the teen to

- Commit to coming to individual and group treatment
- Fill out a diary card (more about this shortly)
- Agree to coaching by phone between sessions
- Learn and practice the DBT skills and whatever other new behaviors are required to live more effectively

This all has to be hammered out before treatment can begin.

Some of you might be thinking that your kid just wouldn't agree to these conditions, or at least not in a meaningful way. It has been my personal experience and the experience of my colleagues, however, that when managed skillfully, adolescents see the value in changing their behavior and will make the commitment. Getting a commitment to therapy, which includes a clear agreement about what behaviors are going to be addressed, as well as specifically what the adolescent will need to do in the therapy, is especially important for kids who are emotionally vulnerable. They are at high risk for dropping out of treatment or for going through the motions without actually making any changes.

The reason has to do with the nature of therapy itself. In therapy the expectation is that one speaks about one's problems, including emotionally difficult ones. Emotionally vulnerable kids tend either to become dysregulated by the discussion and avoid therapy (i.e., drop out) or they're going to speak only about the most bland and often less relevant issues in their lives as a way to avoid becoming emotionally overwhelmed. Getting a real commitment about what work the DBT therapy is going to entail helps prepare the child for what's coming down the pike. The therapist's commitment to help teens with their emotionally dysregulated behavior through skills training and coaching provides them with the invaluable feeling that they will not be alone on this journey. All too

> When the proper initial work isn't done to get an understanding and a commitment from adolescents, they embark on the voyage with the therapist without a shared map.

often when this work is not initially done, the therapist and the child embark on a therapeutic voyage without a shared map. One great way to be sure they're sharing a map is for the adolescent to use a special daily log called a "diary card."

Diary Cards

"Can I see your diary card? What is on your agenda for today?" I asked Shannon.

"Let's see, I have it in my bag somewhere. Oh, here it is," Shannon said as she rummaged through her backpack. "I need to tell you about the fight I had with my boyfriend, Alex. He was just a jerk. I don't know why I even hang out with him. You will never believe what he did," she added as she handed me the diary card.

"Okay, so we need to talk about the fight with Alex. Hold on a minute—you cut yourself on Thursday, so we absolutely need to have that on the agenda for today. I don't remember my pager going off on Thursday," I said in a casual way. "So we are also going to have to talk about why you didn't page me," I added.

The simplest kind of diary card is a grid that has the identified target behaviors along the top of the card and the days of the week going down its left-hand side (see pages 108–109). Each box in the grid is cut in half along the diagonal, and the bottom half has a Y or an N in it representing either Yes or No in response to whether the teen engaged in that specific target. In the top half of the grid she's asked to rate the highest urge to engage in the behavior on that particular day. The back of the diary card lists all the DBT skills, and she is asked to circle which ones she practiced on each day. Some DBT therapists use a more complicated diary card that monitors more emotions and behaviors (see pages 110–111).

DIARY CARD

Target Behaviors						
Monday	1 2 3 4 5 / Yes No	1 2 3 4 5 / Yes No	1 2 3 4 5 / Yes No	1 2 3 4 5 / Yes No	1 2 3 4 5 / Yes No	1 2 3 4 5 / Yes No
Tuesday	1 2 3 4 5 / Yes No	1 2 3 4 5 / Yes No	1 2 3 4 5 / Yes No	1 2 3 4 5 / Yes No	1 2 3 4 5 / Yes No	1 2 3 4 5 / Yes No
Wednesday	1 2 3 4 5 / Yes No	1 2 3 4 5 / Yes No	1 2 3 4 5 / Yes No	1 2 3 4 5 / Yes No	1 2 3 4 5 / Yes No	1 2 3 4 5 / Yes No
Thursday	1 2 3 4 5 / Yes No	1 2 3 4 5 / Yes No	1 2 3 4 5 / Yes No	1 2 3 4 5 / Yes No	1 2 3 4 5 / Yes No	1 2 3 4 5 / Yes No
Friday	1 2 3 4 5 / Yes No	1 2 3 4 5 / Yes No	1 2 3 4 5 / Yes No	1 2 3 4 5 / Yes No	1 2 3 4 5 / Yes No	1 2 3 4 5 / Yes No
Saturday	1 2 3 4 5 / Yes No	1 2 3 4 5 / Yes No	1 2 3 4 5 / Yes No	1 2 3 4 5 / Yes No	1 2 3 4 5 / Yes No	1 2 3 4 5 / Yes No
Sunday	1 2 3 4 5 / Yes No	1 2 3 4 5 / Yes No	1 2 3 4 5 / Yes No	1 2 3 4 5 / Yes No	1 2 3 4 5 / Yes No	1 2 3 4 5 / Yes No

Rate urges or feelings on a scale of 1–5. Circle Yes or No to indicated presence of behavior.

(cont.)

DIARY CARD (*cont.*)

	M	T	W	Th	F	S	S
Wise Mind: Access wisdom. Know truth. Be centered and calm. Integrate Emotional Mind and Reasonable Mind. Meditate.							
Observe: Just notice the experience. "Teflon Mind." Control your attention. Smell the roses. Experience what is happening.							
Describe: Put experiences into words. Describe what is happening. Put words on the experience, say them in your mind.							
Participate: Enter into the experience. Act intuitively from wise mind. Practice changing the harmful and accepting yourself.							
Nonjudgmental Stance: See but don't evaluate. Unglue your opinions. Accept each moment.							
One-Mindfully: Be in the moment. Do one thing at a time. Let go of distractions. Concentrate your mind on the task at hand.							
Effectiveness: Focus on what works. Learn the rules. Play by the rules. Act skillfully. Let go of vengeances and useless anger.							
Objective Effectiveness: DEAR MAN. Describe. Express. Assert. Reinforce. Mindful. Appear confident. Negotiate.							
Relationship Effectiveness: GIVE. Gentle. Interested. Validation. Easy manner.							
Self-Respect Effectiveness: FAST. Fair. No Apologies. Stick to values. Be Truthful.							
Reduce Vulnerability: PLEASE. Treat PhysicaL illness. Balance Eating. Avoid drugs. Balance Sleep. Exercise daily.							
Build Mastery: Try to do one (hard or challenging) thing a day to make yourself feel competent and in control.							
Build Positive Experiences: Do pleasant things. Be mindful of positive experiences. Be unmindful of worries.							
Opposite to Emotion Action: Change emotions by acting opposite to current emotion. Approach rather than avoid.							
Distract: Wise Mind ACCEPTS. Activities. Contributing. Comparisons. Emotions. Pushing away. Thoughts. Senses.							
Self-Soothe: With the five senses. Sights, sounds, smells, tastes, and touch. Be mindful of soothing sensations.							
IMPROVE the Moment: Imagery. Meaning. Prayer. Relaxation. One thing in the moment. Vacation. Encouragement.							
Pros and Cons: Think about the +/− aspects of tolerating distress. Think of the +/− of not tolerating distress.							
Radical Acceptance: Choose to recognize and accept reality. Acceptance does not have to mean approval. Commit to Acceptance = Turning the Mind.							

Dialectical Behavior Therapy **Adolescent Diary Card**	**First name**					**Filled out in session?** Yes/no		

Date	Self-harm		Suicidal		Alcohol		Drugs		Meds
	Urge	Actions	Thoughts	Actions	Urge	Use amount/ type	Urge	Use amount/ type	Taken as prescribed
	0–5	Yes/no	0–5	Yes/no	0–5		0–5		Yes/no

*USED SKILLS

0 = Not thought about or used	4 = Tried, could do them, but they didn't help
1 = Thought about, not used, didn't want to	5 = Tried, could use them, helped
2 = Thought about, not used, wanted to	6 = Didn't try, used them, didn't help
3 = Tried but couldn't use them	7 = Didn't try, used them, helped

Instructions: Circle the days you worked on each skill.

Core Mindfulness	1. Wise mind	Mon	Tues	Wed	Thur	Fri	Sat	Sun
	2. Observe (Just notice what's going on inside)	Mon	Tues	Wed	Thur	Fri	Sat	Sun
	3. Describe (Put words on the experience)	Mon	Tues	Wed	Thur	Fri	Sat	Sun
	4. Participate (Enter into the experience)	Mon	Tues	Wed	Thur	Fri	Sat	Sun
	5. Don't judge (Nonjudgmental stance)	Mon	Tues	Wed	Thur	Fri	Sat	Sun
	6. Stay focused (One-mindfully: in the moment)	Mon	Tues	Wed	Thur	Fri	Sat	Sun
	7. Do what works (Effectiveness)	Mon	Tues	Wed	Thur	Fri	Sat	Sun
Emotion Regulation	8. Identifying and labeling emotions	Mon	Tues	Wed	Thur	Fri	Sat	Sun
	9. PLEASE (Reduce vulnerability to emotion mind)	Mon	Tues	Wed	Thur	Fri	Sat	Sun
	10. MASTER (Building mastery, feeling effective)	Mon	Tues	Wed	Thur	Fri	Sat	Sun
	11. Engaging in pleasant activities	Mon	Tues	Wed	Thur	Fri	Sat	Sun
	12. Working toward long-term goals	Mon	Tues	Wed	Thur	Fri	Sat	Sun
	13. Building structure / time, work, play	Mon	Tues	Wed	Thur	Fri	Sat	Sun
	14. Acting opposite to current emotion	Mon	Tues	Wed	Thur	Fri	Sat	Sun

From Miller, A. L., Rathus, J. H., & Linehan, M. M. (2007). *Dialectical behavior therapy with suicidal adolescents.* Copyright 2007 by The Guilford Press. Reprinted by permission.

How often did you fill out this section? ___ Daily ___ 2–3x ___ Once												Date started
How often did you use phone consult? ___												
Other				Emotions								Notes:
Cut class/ school	Risky sex			Anger	Fear	Happy	Anxious	Sad	Shame	Misery	Skills*	
Yes/no	Yes/no			0–5	0–5	0–5	0–5	0–5	0–5	0–5	0–7	

Rating scale for emotions and urges (above):

0 = Not at all   1 = A bit   2 = Somewhat   3 = Rather strong   4 = Very strong   5 = Extremely strong

Urge to quit therapy: _____   Misery index: _____

Instructions: Circle the days you worked on each skill.

Interpersonal Effectiveness	15. DEAR MAN (Getting what you want)	Mon	Tues	Wed	Thur	Fri	Sat	Sun
	16. GIVE (Improving the relationship)	Mon	Tues	Wed	Thur	Fri	Sat	Sun
	17. FAST (Feeling effective and keeping your self-respect)	Mon	Tues	Wed	Thur	Fri	Sat	Sun
	18. Cheerleading statements for worry thoughts	Mon	Tues	Wed	Thur	Fri	Sat	Sun
Distress Tolerance	19. ACCEPTS (Distract)	Mon	Tues	Wed	Thur	Fri	Sat	Sun
	20. Self-soothe (Five senses)	Mon	Tues	Wed	Thur	Fri	Sat	Sun
	21. Pros and cons	Mon	Tues	Wed	Thur	Fri	Sat	Sun
	22. Radical acceptance	Mon	Tues	Wed	Thur	Fri	Sat	Sun
Walking the Middle Path	23. Positive reinforcement	Mon	Tues	Wed	Thur	Fri	Sat	Sun
	24. Validate self	Mon	Tues	Wed	Thur	Fri	Sat	Sun
	25. Validate someone else	Mon	Tues	Wed	Thur	Fri	Sat	Sun
	26. Think dialectically (not in black and white)	Mon	Tues	Wed	Thur	Fri	Sat	Sun
	27. Act dialectically (walk the middle path)	Mon	Tues	Wed	Thur	Fri	Sat	Sun

The Therapist as Juggler

Setting the stage for therapy with an adolescent is like being a juggler who has to keep his eyes on three crystal balls—one slipup and you've got glass shards at your feet. The first ball is the relationship ball. I want to make sure that the child and I are going to be a good enough match. I know that our relationship is going to be tested from time to time, and I want to have some confidence that we're going to like and have sufficient respect for each other when the going gets tough.

The second ball has to do with the goal of therapy: What does the teen want to change, and what is his or her current level of commitment to the process? Am I going to have to do a fair amount of commitment work or is this patient ready to make some changes? As a DBT therapist I am actively trying to stretch these teens to get them to commit to stopping self-injury and I'm willing to settle for the best they can do in the moment. So while I would like to get them to commit taking self-injury off the table for good, I will settle for less and keep working over time to firm up the commitment.

Finally, the third ball has to do with the external context in which the child lives. For example, are the parents supportive of therapy? Is the child in a school setting that is going to tolerate some behavioral ups and downs? In the beginning of therapy, especially DBT, all these factors are discussed with an eye on how they may play out in the future.

MATTHEW: UNDERSTANDING HOW
THE PROBLEM DEVELOPED

As I've mentioned before, children who engage in self-harming behaviors generally see themselves as weak and/or defective. They believe that if they were stronger or had more willpower, they wouldn't be so overwhelmed by their emotions. I have also met some children who don't think there's anything wrong with self-harming since it helps them feel better and doesn't hurt anyone else. This rationale usually develops because the child has given up any hope of stopping the behavior.

As we've discussed, the legacy of your teen's inability to effectively manage his or her emotional life includes poor self-esteem, depressed mood, a flimsy sense of identity, and a tendency toward impulsive behavior. Trying to reason a kid out of the position that he cuts because he has a character flaw is about as productive as shoveling sand to keep the tide from coming in. The solution instead is to offer a different explanation for the behavior, one that resonates with his experience. In DBT that alternative is the biosocial theory. I like to explain this theory to the teen and the parent in the same session in order to get everybody engaged in the work, as I did with Matthew.

"I have really tried to stop, but nobody believes me. My parents tell me that if I truly wanted to, I would just stop. I know my father thinks I am a weakling for doing it," Matthew bemoaned. "Maybe he's right. I obviously haven't tried hard enough because I'm still doing it."

"So, like your dad, you sometimes think that the problem is a lack of willpower or self-discipline," I replied. "Not only is that theory probably untrue, but it guarantees that you will continue feeling lousy about yourself. From what you've told me about how hard you work in school and manage all those extracurricular activities, you don't strike me as someone who is short on willpower or discipline," I added. "I think there may be a more accurate explanation. Are you interested in hearing about it?"

"Okay," he replied half-heartedly.

"Great, but first I have to ask you three questions. When you think about yourself compared to other people you know, do you think you are more sensitive?" I asked.

"Absolutely!" was his immediate reply.

"Okay. As you think about yourself, do you notice that your emotional reaction time is really quick? That is, you're not someone who has to ponder your feelings—your response is almost immediate."

"Yeah, I think that's true for me. Although sometimes I don't know what I feel, I'm just overwhelmed by emotions."

"All right. Do you think it takes you longer to calm down than other people when you get emotionally revved up?" I asked.

"Most definitely. My dad is always telling me to get over it already. But it's not so easy for me," Matthew said.

"I think your dad may have a hard time understanding that you experience your emotions very differently than he does. So here is my best guess about you. I think you're someone we would call an emotionally reactive person. That means you're hard-wired to feel things in a more powerful way than the average person. In and of itself this is not a psychological problem. The world is full of sensitive people. They are often artists or writers or even shrinks. We need sensitive people. It only becomes a problem when we haven't developed the skills to manage our high-powered emotional systems. When we don't have those skills we are emotionally vulnerable. From what you have told me about your dad, he seems to be the kind of person who operates more on the logical and rational side of things, while you're more about the emotional side of life. Do I have that right?" I wondered.

"For sure. My dad is a computer scientist and I want to be a poet. Sometimes I think we just don't speak the same language," he replied.

"I wouldn't be surprised if your father had a hard time accepting your way of experiencing your feelings. He may have tried to talk you out of what you were feeling or suggested that you were overreacting. At any rate, he probably had a hard time validating your emotional experience. I don't know how your mom fits into this picture because we haven't spoken about her much, but it would be useful to also think about her response to you. I bet you and your parents were doing the best you could, but for a variety of reasons just missed some things in helping you learn how to manage that powerful emotional system of yours."

As you can see, the biosocial theory offers adolescents an alternative explanation for their troubles that resonates with their personal experience—it makes sense according to their view of themselves. It's also a first step in undercutting their deeply held and painful notion that they're weak or defective. Furthermore, the theory leads directly into the primary goal of the treatment: to help them build a useful skill base from which to manage their emotions effectively.

> *The biosocial theory is a powerful way to help adolescents (1) view their self-harming behavior in a new light, (2) let go of the deeply held and painful notion that they are weak or defective, and (3) build a useful skill base from which to manage their emotions effectively.*

David's story illustrates the third goal in the early phase of therapy: figuring out whether patient and therapist are a good match and stressing the importance of open communication.

DAVID: IT'S A MATCH

The week before, my conversation with 17-year-old David had focused on getting him to begin to understand the function of his cutting and to assess his long- and short-term goals, and reviewing the biosocial theory. At the end of the session I suggested that he take some time to think about whether what we had spoken about made sense and whether he was willing to make the commitment to tackle the problem. In our second meeting I began to outline what would be required of him and what would be required of me. With this solid foundation, the therapy to follow would have a much greater chance of succeeding. My job was to balance the seriousness of this process with a light touch.

"Welcome back! Have you thought about what we talked about last week?" I asked David.

"Yeah, a little bit. I don't know. It seems like a lot of work, and I've been in therapy a whole bunch of times and, no offense, but I think it is mostly B.S. Just talking about my problems doesn't seem to help me," David replied.

"Well, I'm not surprised by that. Just talking about your problems doesn't usually help someone like you. In fact, some kids tell me it makes them even worse. As I mentioned last week, we're going to have to get you to do some things differently. So let's talk about your problems and I'll help you learn new skills to manage your life more effectively. You and I will agree on the behaviors you want to change—called "target behaviors"—and we'll work specifically on those. How does that sound?" I answered.

"Well, I really have to get myself together, and soon. I want to go off to school next year, and my parents aren't going to let me go unless I stop cutting. And you know, I don't think cutting is helping me, except in the short run. So I guess I've got nothing to lose."

"Okay. From what you can tell so far, do you think you and I are a good match to work together?" I asked. "The reason I ask is that we have to really be able to collaborate, and if I'm doing things that are annoying you, you have to be able to let me know; and if you're doing something that is interfering with the therapy, I have to be honest with you about it."

DBT requires both the therapist and the patient to sign off on some clearly articulated agreements. We know the treatment is most likely going to have some rocky moments, and we want to do all we can to guard against kids dropping out. We can't help patients if they don't show up, or if all they do is show up and not participate in a meaningful way.

"I think we can work together. So far I have felt pretty comfortable with you," David said.

"Terrific! I know I'm giving you a lot of information about the therapy, but it's important for you to truly understand what you're getting into. This is going to be hard work, and I understand you have a kind of deadline to get this done in time for school next year," I replied.

"Absolutely! I can't wait to get done with high school and get off to college. I need to get on with my life!" David replied enthusiastically.

"All right, then. I'm going to tell you what you can expect from me and then what I expect from you, okay? I am going to do my job to the best of my ability. I am going to meet with you regularly and do everything in my power to help you meet your goals. I'm good at what I do, but I sometimes need help.

You should know that I'm part of a team of therapists who meet weekly to talk about our patients. If I think I'm losing my way, or if you think that I'm not being helpful, then I will get consultation from my team. Have I explained this clearly? Good. Now I'm going to explain what I expect of you.

"First, you need to attend both individual therapy and skills group for 6 months. That seems to be the right amount of time to get what we need to get done. Second, I expect that you will learn and *practice* the DBT skills. This is key. Learning the skills is important, but practicing them in real life is essential. Just learning the skills is like learning to play the piano in music theory class without putting your fingers on the keys. In agreeing to be in therapy with me, you are committing to work on stopping your self-injurious behavior. I also expect that you will fill out your diary card on a daily basis and bring it with you to our sessions. Finally, if you're feeling bad and have tried some skills, but you're still thinking of hurting yourself, you have to page me."

"Page you?" David asked. "You mean anytime, 24/7?"

"Yes, anytime, day or night," I responded. "What do you think would get in the way of your doing it?" I inquired.

"I don't know. I wouldn't want to bother you with my problems in the middle of the night. And anyway, I just have to learn how to deal."

"You are absolutely going to have to get better at dealing with your problems, David. I couldn't agree more. That's why you need my help with skills coaching when you're in the midst of a crisis. Think about it this way: I'm like the orchestra conductor and you're my orchestra. The conductor and the orchestra meet regularly for rehearsals—that's our therapy. The actual concert is real life, what happens outside this office. Now, can you imagine a conductor only being available for practice and not for the performance?" I explained. "I'm not crazy about being awakened in the middle of the night, but I much prefer that to being useless as your therapist."

> *Learning the DBT skills is important, and practicing them in real life is even more important. Just learning the skills is like learning to play the piano in music theory class without putting your fingers on the keys.*

"Okay. When you explain it that way, I see your point," David replied.

The telephone skills-coaching sessions are sometimes hard for kids to understand at first, but they can offer exactly the right help when the urge to harm overcomes them after they've tried the skills I've been teaching them. Stephanie's story is a good illustration.

STEPHANIE:
A TELEPHONE SKILLS-COACHING SESSION

My pager goes off just after midnight on Saturday. It's Stephanie, a 16-year-old girl who has been in DBT treatment with me for about 3 months.

"I feel terrible," she tells me through tears. "I really want to cut. I know it will make me feel better. I just can't stand it anymore. I hate my boyfriend! He is just a real S.O.B. You can't believe what he did to me."

"You sound really upset. I know that boyfriend of yours can be really insensitive. Tell me, before you paged me, what skills did you try to help you regain your balance?" I asked.

"I tried some interpersonal effective skills with him, but he just blew me off. I even wrote out what I wanted to say, and he just didn't give a damn. I just want to hurt myself. I hate him so much." She sobbed into the phone. "I don't know what to do."

"Well, you did the right thing by paging me before you cut. Good for you! It seems to me that right now what's most important is getting you safely through this crisis. Which of the crisis survival skills has been helpful in the past?" I asked.

"I don't know! I'm so angry. I don't care what happens to me. He's the one who—"

"Stephanie," I interrupted, "you called me for help. I can give it to you, but it doesn't involve talking about your boyfriend right now. We've talked in session about the self-soothing skills that work best for you. Which ones might be good to try right now?"

"Ummm, I guess I could put on my headphones and listen to my music, especially the upbeat stuff," Stephanie replied.

"Okay. What might you try after that?"

"I could take a shower and put on my flannel pj's. I'm going to turn off my phone because I'm not going to talk to my boyfriend anymore tonight or I'd cut for sure," she said, clearly starting to calm down.

"Great! You're starting to think of ways to help yourself get through these difficult feelings without making it worse. Terrific job! I would love to get a voice mail at my office letting me know how the night worked out for you."

"Yeah, I can do that. Thanks, Doc. I will leave you a message," she said.

One of the most effective aspects of DBT is the between-session skills coaching. Stephanie and countless other patients would have harmed themselves without it. Later that night she left a voice mail for me saying how she'd listened to some music and taken a shower before settling down to sleep—with her phone turned off. In DBT adolescents are *required* to access their individual therapists, day or night, if they are about to engage in what they've identified as target behaviors. First, the teens should try their new skills to manage the crisis. If that doesn't work, they should page the therapist. In the very beginning of treatment, before they've been exposed to the DBT skills, paging before trying a skill is reasonable. After a short while, however, it's important for them to try their skills before paging. Paging is not psychotherapy over the phone; it is limited to a quick assessment of the situation (including a suicide assessment, if warranted) and then skills coaching.

What's your role in all this? The answer will be hard to hear: little or none. Once you're aware that your child is struggling, you naturally want to encourage him to call the therapist. Your anxiety level is high, and in all likelihood your child is becoming emotionally dysregulated. The scene is set for a discussion that is going to be emotionally charged and quickly go off track. My advice is to gently remind the child that the therapist is available to him. At the next meeting, the issue is probably going to come up. If the child did not page, he and the therapist will figure out why not and what they can do next time to make sure he pages when he's in crisis.

There's more: The therapist can't let you in on everything that goes on in the weekly sessions and the between-sessions coaching.

MY POLICY ON CONFIDENTIALITY

The following occurred in the second meeting I had with Manny and his mother, Isabella.

"Now that Manny and I have agreed to work together and we have some clear ideas about what needs to change, I thought we should discuss issues around confidentiality," I said. "It's important that we all understand what and how information is going to be shared."

"I don't want to know every detail of what you talk about in therapy, but if he hurts himself I would like to know," Manny's mom replied.

"It makes sense that you would want to know, and my worry is that my telling you is likely to make it more difficult for Manny to honestly tell me what is going on. Here's what I propose: if I don't think we're making progress on this issue, then we will all meet to see what we can figure out. How does that sound?" I asked.

"All right, but I do worry that he's going to really hurt himself badly," Isabella said.

"If I think that Manny is at risk for seriously hurting himself, then I will not hesitate to call you and to take whatever measures are necessary to prevent him from doing that," I said. "Are you clear about that, Manny?"

"Yeah, but I'm not going to do anything stupid," he said.

"Great! Now I want your mom to know that she can call me and give me information anytime she wants. Here's the deal, however: whenever she calls I will always let you know what she told me. So, Isabella, I suggest that if you're going to call, you let Manny know. And that you understand that I will be speaking with Manny about your concerns," I said.

"Okay. I like the idea that I can call you if I'm worried," she replied.

"Yes, you can. Of course our goal would be for you and Manny to have that conversation," I said.

I routinely bring up the issue of confidentiality in the first or second session. This discussion needs to include the teen, the parents, and any other mental health professionals in the child's life. I make sure I am clear with everyone involved about what they can expect me to share and what I am going to keep confidential. Breaking confidentiality is more complex than just deciding it's warranted if suicide or harm to others seem possible. It also has to do with the patient's age and stage of development. For example, a 13-year-old found drinking alcohol is a different story than an 18-year-old doing the same thing. A certain amount of privacy is crucial in order for the treatment to proceed effectively.

There is a fine line, however, between age-appropriate privacy and secrecy that undercuts the therapy. For example, it's a problem for a therapist to know that a kid is smoking marijuana on a daily basis and to keep that from you for the long term—it's bound to undercut your confidence in the therapist and potentially minimize the damaging aspect of the behavior on your child. Generally, I do not break confidentiality if my patient engages in self-harm. I certainly can empathize with parents' wish to know. But in my experience, divulging such behavior is all too often counterproductive: it can make the adolescent clam up about it in the therapy.

Therapists may vary in their rules about keeping your child's harmful behavior from you, but in general:

1. They will let you know if a suicide attempt appears to be a real threat.
2. They will not let you know if an act of self-injury is revealed to them.
3. They will let you know if therapy is not progressing.

YOUR THERAPIST'S POLICY
ON CONFIDENTIALITY

Ask the therapist directly and get a clear understanding about what informa-tion he or she will share with you and when. Trying to determine the balance between how much information you need to have and how much privacy your child needs to make effective use of the therapy is extremely difficult for the therapist.

One hard-and-fast rule is that if the therapist thinks the child is in dan-ger of suicide, then he or she must break confidentiality. But most deliberate self-harm is not about suicide, and breaking confidentiality when the patient engages in the behavior may seriously compromise the therapy. On the other hand, keeping parents in the dark about the behavior for too long risks under-mining their confidence in the treatment. The good news here is that this is a resolvable dilemma.

One of the biggest challenges for the therapist, especially in the begin-ning of a therapy, is to determine whether the kid's wish for confidentiality is in the service of keeping a secret or whether it is an expression of the need for a private space to understand and examine his or her behavior. Most adoles-cents experience some degree of shame around self-injury that pushes them in the direction of hiding it. Furthermore, adolescents worry about how their parents will respond to deliberate self-harm and whether their friends will truly understand.

In addition, there may be strong consequences for the child if his or her behavior comes to the attention of school administrators, including being re-quired to take a medical leave until the situation is remedied. If the adoles-cent is committed to ending self-injury and is actively engaged in treatment, then from my point of view he is entitled to a degree of privacy. If, however, he has made only a half-hearted commitment to the therapy and is frequently not following through on treatment requirements, then I think it is time to reexamine the therapy, including issues of confidentiality.

So you need to understand that it's not wise to share with you everything that happens in your child's therapy. This brings up the topic of the match be-tween you and the therapist and how you can be of the most help to your child.

THERAPISTS AND PARENTS

Most therapists and parents find ways to work together. Occasionally, how-ever, the contact between parents and therapist is problematic, even though the parents and the therapist feel that this is the right match. These problems do not have to stand in the way of effective therapy if you keep the following ideas in mind.

First, each party might be coming to the table with a fair amount of emotional freight. The very idea that they have a child in need of treatment makes some parents feel that they've failed in some way. The guilt and shame around this misguided idea can be a fertile ground for defensive and aloof behavior.

As for the therapist, he or she may feel inadequate when parents raise concerns for which there are no clear answers. We just don't know enough to respond definitively to questions about the outcome of the treatment. Furthermore, individuals vary a lot in their response to treatment.

Some therapists can be defensive. We can sometimes be distracted by the intensity of your fear and anxiety, forgetting that this is a perfectly understandable response to a child's dysfunction. Instead of allaying your fears with clear answers, we often have to ask you to be patient. Therapy is not an exact science.

Therapists are only human, and we can be influenced by how we are treated. What makes me as a therapist eager to respond to parents' questions has a lot to do with their attitude. I tend to respond more positively to parents who appear genuinely curious about the process of therapy and who, even if they feel it, do not openly express skepticism. Parents who are actively interested in collaboration are always going to get my best.

Here's an example of an ineffective comment from a parent: "So what makes you think you can be helpful to our daughter?"

And an effective one: "Help me understand how you're going to be helpful to our daughter."

Both comments occur after an explanation of how therapy works, but the first is adversarial. The second is more of an invitation. Think of yourself as being on the same team with the therapist, a coaching team that is going to help your child learn and practice being in the world in a different way.

All the elements I'm discussing in this chapter form a piece of the puzzle that, when completed, will yield some workable solutions to your child's troubles. One step leads to another in a chain, which we refer to as a "chain analysis." As I continued to talk with Shannon, a chain analysis of her target behavior began to emerge. In other words, together we began to see what triggered her to cut and what specific tools would give her the capacity to stop.

SHANNON: "I'M READY TO TRY SOMETHING ELSE"

"Let's see, Shannon, on Thursday you cut yourself. When did that happen?" I asked.

"I don't know, sometime late Thursday night, I guess. Yeah, it must have been, because I was in my pajamas washing up for bed," she told me.

"Do you remember when the idea first came into your head to cut?" I wondered.

"No. I don't really think I ever thought about it. It just happened. I can't believe what my boyfriend did. First, he calls me and tells me that—"

"You know, I really am interested in what happened between you and your boyfriend, but first we have to figure out the cutting," I interrupted. "What did you do after you hung up the phone?" I asked.

"I went into my room and got into my pajamas to get ready for bed. Then I went into the bathroom to wash up. I was still feeling really mad and hurt. You know, I saw my razor and without really thinking I just started to cut," Shannon said. "I just needed to get some relief."

"When you were getting into your Pj's, were you thinking about hurting yourself?" I inquired.

"Well, now that you mention it, I was just crazy on the inside and just hating my boyfriend and I thought maybe if I cut myself, like I used to, I would feel better. I kind of didn't care about anything. I just wanted some peace," she reported.

"So you first had the thought while you were getting into your pajamas, and it sounds like you were in the kind of mood that you needed just to get some short-term relief from that crazy feeling," I suggested.

"That's right, and there was the razor and I just did it," she told me.

"Okay. Then it seems when you get into that mood, we need to help you find some solutions other than self-injury. We need to find a way to slow you down and help you change your mood so you can think more clearly. I have some ideas about some skills that might be really useful in those moments. What do you think?" I asked.

"I'm ready to try something else. To be honest with you, cutting really only made me feel crappier about myself," she said.

After several chain analyses the patient and I develop a *behavioral analysis*—a relatively comprehensive understanding of the patterns and events that lead to a target behavior. Throughout the various chain analyses the child and I are generating possible solutions that would have avoided the necessity of engaging in a target behavior. In the *solution analysis* we look at all the places in the chain of events where the patient could have made more effective behavioral choices, and specifically what those more effective behaviors might have been. Following that analysis we decide which new skillful behaviors need to be learned and practiced.

FOCUSING ON TARGET BEHAVIORS

You might be asking yourself, How do you know which target behaviors to address in a chain analysis? In DBT there is a hierarchy of target behaviors that guide the therapist. The number one priority is any suicidal or self-harming behaviors. If the adolescent has contemplated suicide, made an attempt, or engaged in deliberate self-harm, or if their urges were high, then a chain analysis of the behavior is a must in the session. Notice in the story with Shannon how she wanted to speak about the fight with her boyfriend, but I was not willing to have that discussion until we had a better understanding of the self-injury. If Shannon had been so emotionally distraught that she had too difficult a time turning her attention to the issue of self-harm, I would have spent more time listening and validating her feelings as a way to get back to looking at the higher target behavior.

BEHAVIOR THAT INTERFERES WITH THERAPY OR QUALITY OF LIFE

The second highest priority is any behavior that interferes with the therapy, such as not filling in the diary card, showing up late for therapy, or refusing to speak about a relevant topic. Therapy-interfering behaviors are not limited to the patient. As a DBT therapist I am always on the alert for anything that I might be doing that is getting in the way of the treatment moving forward. I also have an agreement with patients that if they think I am engaging in therapy-interfering behaviors, they have to let me know, and they usually do.

The third priority deals with behaviors that interfere with quality of life. These are things like skipping school, excessive use of drugs or alcohol, and non-life-threatening eating disorders. When parents are concerned about anything that fits into the category of therapy-interfering behavior, I urge them to give me a call.

SKILLS TRAINING IN ACTION:
LEARNING TO SELF-SOOTHE

"Okay, Shannon, now that we see the pattern about how that awful mood state leads to self-injury, let's go to work on helping you use skills to change your mood," I said.

"All right, but when I get like that, I feel pretty stuck and hopeless," she replied.

"I believe that is all too true, and I know that with some work you will know how to get yourself unstuck from that terrible mood," I replied. "We need to think about a chain of skills. Here is what I am thinking, and I need you to tell me whether this makes sense to you. First let me ask you this: Do you know pretty quickly when you're falling into that black mood?" I asked.

"Not always. Sometimes I realize I am in that mood and that I have been feeling this way for some time."

"All right, then. Here's what I think. You and I figured out earlier that interpersonal conflict—a fight with the boyfriend, troubles with parents—is likely to move you into that mood. What we need to work on is helping you to use some mindfulness skills so that you are able to observe and describe the situation and cue yourself to prepare for the black mood. I know this sounds simple, but at first it's not going to be an easy thing to do. It will take some practice. I think the next step is to move right into some emotion regulation skills and the distress-tolerance crisis survival skills. Do you know which of those skills work for you?" I wondered.

"Yes, believe it or not, I like opposite action to emotion and some of the self-soothing skills," she replied.

"You are the greatest! Which self-soothe works for you? And what action would you use when you're starting to get into that mood?" I asked.

"When I'm in that mood, all I want to do is go to bed and try and forget everything. So opposite action would be doing something active, like going for a walk or even dancing in my room. For self-soothe I have this really great book of impressionist paintings—I could look at that," Shannon told me.

Shannon was making real progress here.

TROUBLESHOOTING

The next step is for Shannon and me to do some trouble shooting about any barriers that would preclude her from using new skills. For example, we might have to anticipate what she should do if her boyfriend calls her, or her father asks her to set the table when she needs some space and is trying to self-soothe. We would also address what to do if something she tries doesn't seem to be working.

As you know, DBT is all about learning the four skill modules. Skills are pushed in during the group therapy and pulled out in the individual therapy: the child learns the skills in the group setting and then the therapist and the patient figure out what skills are called for to help the child manage whatever issues are of concern. DBT skills groups are more like educational seminars than like traditional group psychotherapy.

In multifamily skills groups, both the child and the parents learn the skill sets. In addition these groups undercut the participants' sense of isolation as they work at resolving their own and their family's difficulties. The next section offers ideas on how you can help your child during the therapy.

WHAT CAN YOU DO?:
SUPPORTING THE THERAPY

You are already supporting the treatment with the sacrifices you're making in terms of time and money, so give yourself some credit. The following suggestions are a few other ways in which you can be helpful.

1. Naturally you want to know what's being worked on in your child's therapy—but you're reluctant to intrude. It's important for you to find a balance between these two positions. The typical teenager is usually able to express consternation when she feels a parent is being intrusive, but has more difficulty addressing the problem of not being noticed. Communicate to your child that you have confidence in the process and are interested in a general way about what is being worked on—but that you don't expect to hear all the details. Let her know that you're interested in anything she feels comfortable sharing.

2. If your kid has complaints about the therapy or the therapist, listen, validate, and help her bring the concerns in to the therapist.

3. When you feel the need to contact the therapist yourself, always let your child know. This helps ward off discussions about intrusiveness and parental control that may miss the point.

4. Let your kid know that you understand change can be hard. Praise her when you see progress.

5. Familiarize yourself with the four skill modules discussed in

Chapter 4 so you'll be better able to help your child use them. Do not however, offer this help until you're clear that the child wants it.

I will have more to say about the ways you can be helpful to your child in Chapter 6.

ASSESSING YOUR CHILD'S PROGRESS

It's important for you to be able to assess your child's progress in therapy. Unfortunately, you probably won't always know when your child is engaging in self-injury, so your assessment will have to be made on indirect factors:

1. Set up periodic reviews of the therapy with the therapist.
2. Discreetly chart the incidence of behaviors that indicate whether the child is making progress or not. (E.g., if your child has had a history of emotional outbursts, you could chart how often these occur and see if over 3 or 4 months the trend is in the downward direction. If it is, then you can assume that your child is making progress toward modulating his emotions—a good sign that self-injury may also be on the decline.)
3. Look for signs of other kinds of skillful behavior. Is your kid asking for things in a more effective way? Does she seem better able to accept disappointments? Is she more interested in sharing her experiences with you? Does she seem less mood-dependent?

The best way to make the assessment about progress is to look at several of these elements over time. The idea is to collect information on several be-

---

TREATMENT REALITIES

1. It's critical that you find a therapist who is not only a good fit for your kid but also someone you think you can work with.
2. Therapy takes time. Plan on your child attending treatment for at least a year.
3. Progress is often uneven. Be thankful for the successes and don't panic if things temporarily slip backward.
4. Therapy is likely to cost you in time and money.
5. These kids often have a high therapy dropout rate—it may take several tries to get the right fit.

haviors because that will give you a better picture of what progress is being made. Progress is going to be an up-and-down process, so look for trends. It takes time. You should expect to see some signs of progress within 4 or 5 months of an outpatient DBT.

Now let's turn to a discussion of what you can do to help your child with emotion regulation.

6

resetting the stage

HOW TO HELP YOUR TEEN RESTORE
EMOTION TO ITS PROPER PLACE

Jenny's mom met her husband at the door. "Jenny's been in the bathroom for over half an hour. She went out with Mikela again, and when she came home she had that look in her eye. I think she's in there cutting herself again."

"Damn it! This always happens when she goes out with that Mikela kid. I'm going up there and if I have to, I'll bust the door in!" shouted Jenny's dad. "She has to stop that crazy behavior right now!"

As parents, we are hard-wired as well as socially engineered to be of use to children. When our children accept our help, it usually gives us a sense of competence and a degree of happiness. There's no doubt about it: successful children help us feel we are great parents, and children who are having trouble leave us wondering about our abilities. One of the ways we feel competent and have a tangible sense that we're doing a good job is when our children do well in school or in music, art, or sports. While we know that this was truly our kids' accomplishment, we also know that we had something to do with it, even if it was just to be encouraging.

It's not always the case, but often we feel we were more successful when our children were younger. When adolescence arrives, it's harder to know how to be helpful; if your child has emotional troubles, the situation becomes even murkier. Parenting strategies that were helpful in the past, such as reassurance or direct problem solving, often now lead to an angry or tearful rejection. The difference between a fictional patient named Mary at age 7 and 14 makes my point.

Little Mary, age 7, comes home from school with a frown on her face, tears welling in her eyes, and lips quivering.

"Mary," you say. "What's the matter?"

"My friend Jamie doesn't want to be my friend anymore because I wouldn't share my cupcake with her," Mary tells you as her tears cascade down her cheeks.

"Oh, not to worry. You and Jamie have been friends for so long, I'm sure you'll make up [reassurance]. I have an idea: Why don't we make some more cupcakes and bring some over to Jamie this afternoon?" you suggest [problem solving].

Mary begins to smile. "You are the best mommy in the world!" she tells you.

Big Mary, age 14, comes home from school with a frown on her face, tears welling in her eyes, and lips quivering.

"Mary," you say. "What's the matter?"

"Nothing!" she shoots back at you with anger.

"Hey, I'm just trying to help, and I know something's wrong," you reply as your emotional temperature begins to climb.

"The problem is that Jamie is a bitch, okay? Now leave me alone," she shouts back at you.

"Mary, you and Jamie have been such good friends, I'm sure you'll be able to patch things up" [reassurance], you reply gingerly. "I'm sure if you and she talk about it, you can work it out" [problem solving].

"Screw Jamie! You're an idiot!" Mary screams as she races to her room.

Similar problem, same strategy—but very different results at different ages. When faced with emotional turmoil, parents, like the rest of humankind, usually fall back on a set of behavioral skills that worked for them in the past. It takes some time, a different perspective, and practice to develop a new set of parenting skills. And skill acquisition occurs best in relatively calm situations, not in moments of crisis and high emotional distress. So it's not surprising that you often can't figure out what to do when faced with your emotionally dysregulated kid. Try as you might, you're likely to repeat formerly successful behavioral strategies that just don't work anymore.

WHAT TO DO AND WHY

Having a child who engages in deliberate self-harm is especially challenging. You're keenly aware that your child is struggling emotionally and you can see that her behavior attacks her own body, a body that you have been trying to safeguard since she was an infant. Like Mary's mother, you often find yourself frustrated, annoyed, and plagued by helpless rage. Or else you become ineffectual by pushing too hard to be helpful.

Sometimes as parents the best you can shoot for is not to make the situation worse and hope that you'll find a way to do better the next time around. When you are parenting a child who is emotionally vulnerable and involved with self-harming behavior, the standard set of parenting skills needs to be refined and new ones learned. For example, validation takes on an importance with these children that goes beyond what other kids need. The good news here is that you can learn some new skills that will optimize the chances that you will be helpful to your child.

The skills discussed in this chapter are going to overlap with the skill sets that I am going to teach you about in the next chapters. So my advice is to read Chapters 7 and 8 before you start implementing some of the skills and you'll be surprised at how your child's reaction to you will change.

In addition to teaching you some new skills, or at the very least helping you refine the skills you already have, I will outline some things that parents have found useful in helping their children through these rough waters: how to balance giving your kid reasonable "emotional space" with low-keyed vigilance, for example, or when to actively intervene in your child's life versus when to let "natural" consequences play out. Finally, for the sake of "covering the waterfront," I'll review a few things that people often try that I just don't think are effective.

One important thing to keep in mind as you work on acquiring new parenting skills is that learning new behavior is like turning around an ocean liner—it takes practice, patience, and perseverance. There's just no way it can be done quickly. Psychologists refer to this process as "shaping behavior"—getting the desired behavior or skill down pat through successive approximations or trials. This means deliberately acknowledging your child's efforts and/or your own

> *Learning new behavior is like turning around an ocean liner—it takes practice, patience, and perseverance.*

when your behavior may not be dead-on but is going in the right direction. Praise yourself and your kid when either of you improve. This will reinforce the behavior—that is, it will make it more likely that the new skillful behavior will occur again. Here's an example of what I mean by shaping.

Big Mary, age 14, comes home from school with a frown on her face, tears welling in her eyes, and lips quivering.

"Mary," you say, "What's the matter?"

"Nothing! Just leave me alone," she shoots back at you.

"Okay, but something has definitely gotten under your skin and is troubling you," you reply, maintaining a degree of equanimity [validation].

"Jamie is a bitch! I hate her!" Mary tells you as her voice begins to rise.

"Whoa, she really annoyed you and hurt your feelings," you reply [validation].

"Yes! Now I just want to be alone," Mary shouts as she heads upstairs to her room.

"I'm sure I could help," you say [unsolicited problem solving].

"Nobody can help. Just leave me alone," Mary tells you from halfway up the stairs.

Here Mary's mom does a more effective job of managing the situation than she did in the first example, but she still falls short of helping Mary through her distress. If Mom had told me about these two incidents in consultation about 14-year-old Mary, I would have pointed out a few things for her to consider. First, in the second incident she was able to maintain a relatively calm manner in the face of her child's emotional distress, thus decreasing the likelihood that the situation would escalate. Second, her use of validation seemed to help Mary continue the conversation. Both of these new skillful behaviors demonstrate that Mary's mom is moving in the right direction. Third, she probably goofed a bit by offering problem solving without asking Mary if she wanted some help. Fourth, I would remind Mom that sometimes no matter what you do you may not get the results you want, but that her behavior the second time around was more on target. She is shaping her behavior to be more helpful when her daughter is in emotional distress.

When you're learning new skills, I encourage you to keep the three Ps in mind: practice, patience, and perseverance. They hold the key to helping your child.

Practice

Practice is just working at a new behavior or skill through repetition. Here are a few suggestions.

1. Don't try to learn a million skills at once. Pick out a few that seem particularly relevant and really commit to learning them.

2. Keep the concept of *shaping* in mind—you just want to keep getting more proficient at the skill you're practicing. It takes time, and some days will be better than others.

3. Remember to acknowledge and reward your successes. Doing so will help *reinforce* your new skillful behavior.

4. Finally, practice your new skillful behaviors in relatively neutral and calm situations. You're not likely to pick up new skills when you're in the

midst of a crisis. While it may be true that throwing someone out of a boat may force him to learn how to swim, I can almost guarantee that he won't become an Olympic champ.

Patience

I can hear you now: "You want me to be patient while my child is self-injuring? You can't be serious! Doctor, slip into your pajamas because you must be dreaming."

Well, you do have a choice: you can either be impatient with your child and yourself, suffer, and make the situation worse, or you can find a way to be patient and, in all probability, more helpful.

Being patient is not synonymous with doing nothing. In fact, being patient in stressful times takes enormous effort. Self-validation, acceptance strategies, and distress tolerance are the skill sets required to be "actively" patient. I'll discuss these in detail in Chapter 8.

Perseverance

Sometimes I think perseverance is best captured by the old adage that it doesn't matter how many times you get knocked down; it only matters how many times you get up. You just need to get up one more time than the number of times you have been knocked down. It sounds simple but it's not. There are two main ingredients in being able to persevere. The first is cultivating an attitude of willingness and the second is being mindful to set achievable goals.

> To persevere you need to cultivate an attitude of willingness—accepting the situation as it is and doing what is required—and you need to be mindful in setting achievable goals.

Willingness

Willingness is about directing our energies to doing what our present circumstances require. By contrast, willfulness is spending energy on things like complaining that our situation is unfair or that things just shouldn't be the way they are. Don't confuse willingness as resignation or as some trick to get you to like your current situation. Willingness is just part of accepting the situation as it is and then turning your mind toward doing what is required.

For example, my family is fortunate to have a swimming pool in our backyard. With the unpredictable summer weather in New England, though, the water is often freezing. My wife and kids always used to get a kick out of watching me get in the pool. I would complain, go halfway down the steps, get in, then whine some more about how cold the water was. They would all just jump in and tell me to do the same, and I would tell them they were crazy. I was the epitome of a willful person. I wanted to swim, but I wanted the water to be warmer.

Then about four summers ago, I decided to try a more willing approach to getting in the pool. That is, I accepted that no matter how much I hated cold water, if I wanted to swim, the water I had to swim in would not be warm. On those days when the pool was cold, I just accepted things as they were and waded in without complaint or delay: I became *willing to do what was required* to get in the pool. I'm sure my family misses the old days when they could tease me about my inability to come to terms with an unpleasant reality, but—while I can't say I like cold water—I certainly enjoy the pool much more than I used to.

Setting Achievable Goals

The second ingredient in perseverance has to do with setting realistic goals. Nothing reinforces success like success, and setting achievable goals is one way to help you stay the course. Let's face it: it's hard to keep going when we experience defeat and failure at every turn. Think about taking small steps toward your goals. For example, if you're working on validation, decide in advance how many times per day or per week you're going to deliberately practice it. This is a small step and a realistic goal. The idea is to build on your small steps and avoid overwhelming defeats.

Practice, patience, and perseverance are the mind-set you need to keep on moving down the rocky path that will enable you to bring help to your child. "It don't come easy," as the song says, so acknowledge your successes and learn from your missteps.

WHAT *NOT* TO DO AND WHY

Before launching into what you can do to be helpful to your child, I'd like to tell you about some things that I don't think work. Some clinicians are still advocating some of these strategies. If what I'm telling you goes against the advice you're currently being given, then I've put you in a tough spot. It could be that these techniques work in your specific situation. If that's the case, I know you'll have the good sense to ignore what I have to say in this instance. If, on the other hand, you're doing some of these things and not getting results, then by all means take it up with the treatment team.

Removing the Tools Your Child Could Use to Self-Injure

It might seem to make sense to hide or rid your house of all the sharp objects your child might use to self-injure. But I think it's a bad idea for at least three reasons. First, there are an infinite number of things she could use, so it's virtually impossible to make the house "safe" and keep it that way for any reasonable period of time. Second, it forces you into the role of constantly policing the house and potentially into an adversarial role with your child. I can see no real advantage in becoming the "sharps police."

Finally, it's far more important for your child to learn how to accommodate to the world as it is—with razors, scissors, knives, pop-tops, and safety pins, to name just a few dangers—than for you to create (even if you could) an artificially "safe" environment. This is a strategy that more often than not lulls parents into a false sense that they're in control of their child's self-injurious behavior. I have heard of more than one situation where well-intended parents have locked up all the sharp objects and the child either found a way to get them or brought new ones into the house.

Don't get me wrong—I'm not suggesting that you leave sharp objects like X-Acto knives or box cutters lying around. Therapists working with kids who engage in self-harming behavior also need to make sure their charges don't have a stash of sharp objects in their rooms or backpacks. I believe that a top priority in treatment is to help teens see the wisdom in not holding on to objects they have used for self-harm and to enlist their help in removing objects of temptation. Please ask your child's therapist how he or she thinks about this issue.

Body Checks

Parents, therapists, and school administrators sometimes request that a kid known to have self-harmed be seen by a medical professional on a regular basis to be examined for fresh evidence. The goal is to know if the kid is still self-injuring, as well as to use the knowledge of upcoming examinations as a deterrent. I have never understood the reasoning behind this strategy. For one thing, asking teenagers to undress and be examined for cuts is going to bring shame and humiliation on them. In the language of behavioral psychology, it's much closer to a punishment than to a reinforcement strategy (as encouraging more skillful behavior would be).

I have no doubt that for some kids the threat of a shameful body check is enough to stop their self-injury. But once the body checks stop, there is a high probability that these kids will go right back to self-injuring. Furthermore, it's not a foolproof procedure, since a body check is usually done with the kid in undergarments, making it possible to hide some injuries. I can't imagine any therapeutic gain from a strategy that is potentially humiliating, nor do I think forcing a child to be more secretive about self-harm is working in the right direction.

So much for the strategies that I think don't work. Now let's talk about the ones that do.

WHAT WORKS AND WHY

Validation

I've talked about validation before. It's probably the single most important skill I can teach you. Validating your child's emotional experience, whether or not you think he or she *should* be having that experience, provides the bridge you need to connect with your child in all kinds of stormy situations. Kids who are emotionally vulnerable probably need more validation than other kids do. They need to learn that their emotional reactions make sense, even when their current strategies for managing these reactions are ineffective. Validation often "sets the table" for an effective collaboration between you and your child.

You will recall that validating your child's experience or point of view is not the same as approving or agreeing; it only acknowledges that you have heard and understood what he's saying with words or body language. Remembering to stay curious and open about how your child is thinking and feeling, even when you believe you have a quick or easy solution, is a challenge for most parents. We want to help and we believe, sometimes correctly, that we have the answers. Or we're frightened for our child and we want him to stop something dangerous, but teens must come to their own wisdom—finding their own way is one of the primary tasks of adolescence.

Validation is kind of quirky. One of the things I have learned is that when parents begin to practice validation, it often sounds artificial and stilted—kind of phony. This is to be expected. Think back to when you first started learning a foreign language or trying to ride a bicycle. When you're learning any new skill, your attempts are going to be anything but smooth. Furthermore, what you say in an effort to be validating is only validating if the person feels it is. If your daughter is revved up after an embarrassing scene at school and you try to validate her, your comments could be spot-on but she could still reject what you say because she just can't take it in. When that happens (and I can almost guarantee it will), don't give up! Just try to understand that the moment wasn't right for your kid to feel validated.

There are several different ways to validate your child's experience, from what we call "attentive listening" to those rare but lovely moments when some action of yours is experienced simultaneously as communicating your understanding of your child's predicament and as comforting. You've had these moments in the past, and as you learn the new skills you need, you'll find them occurring more often. In this chapter I'm going to concentrate on three different types of validation that I have found to be the easiest for parents to learn and that really work. But before I get into the details of these validation strategies, I want to bring up some pitfalls.

Don't Validate the Invalid

It is ineffective to validate what is patently not valid, as Robert's mother tries to do.

"I can't believe how stupid I am! I stayed up all night studying for my advance placement history test and I still got a C–. I am just the dumbest kid in my school," Robert said as he choked back tears.

"You may be the dumbest kid in your school, but your father and I still love you," Robert's mother replied in her most gentle voice.

Here are some other ways that Robert's mother could have responded, rather than validate Robert's feeling that he's stupid: "After all that hard work, it is really disheartening to get a low grade," or "I can see how you might doubt your abilities when you get a grade like that," or even "I can understand how you might think you're dumb when you get a C– on a test for which you had prepared."

Avoid Personal References

"I can't believe Jane would treat me this way! I thought we were best friends and then she goes and betrays me like this. I'm going to make her pay," Elizabeth said through clenched teeth.

"I know exactly how you feel," her mother replied. "When I was your age, the same thing happened to me with my best friend."

"Who cares? I don't want to hear about it. Just leave me alone," Elizabeth angrily replied.

You may very well have had experiences that are similar to what your child is facing, and you may very well have managed them in ways that could be helpful to your child. The problem is that when you introduce your own experience into the discussion, the scale tips toward you and away from your kid. Validation is all about communicating an understanding of the *other* person's experience.

Your past experiences can be useful, however, so here's one way you can both validate your child and speak about your own experiences.

"I can't believe Jane would treat me this way! I thought we were best friends and then she goes and betrays me like this. I'm going to make her pay," Elizabeth said through clenched teeth.

"You're really mad! What did Elizabeth do that got you so angry and hurt?" Elizabeth's mom asked.

"I don't want to talk about it," Elizabeth shot back.

"Okay. Are you just too mad right now?" Elizabeth's mom inquired.

"Yeah. I don't know how she could just disregard me like she did. I told her not to tell anybody about being in the hospital, and then she goes and tells Cheryl. What's up with that?" Elizabeth said.

"That's awful! No wonder you're mad," Mom replied. "If at some point you want to talk about it, I can tell you about what I did when a good friend betrayed me."

"Sure, Mom, but not right now," Elizabeth replied.

In this case Elizabeth's mom does a fair amount of validating before offering help. The validation is in the service of understanding and being supportive of Elizabeth. Validation often seems to invite the other person to talk more about the problem. Elizabeth tells her mother more in spite of just having said that she doesn't want to talk about the situation. Please notice that before offering her daughter help, the mom asks whether Elizabeth wants it. This is important! In general, but especially with adolescents, unsolicited advice is experienced as intrusive and unwelcome. Kids will often experience it as a sign that you don't believe they can manage their own problems, so it feels like being kicked when they're down. When you ask your kid whether she wants your advice, you are maximizing the probability that she will listen to what you have to say. Don't waste the wisdom you have earned over the years by offering it too early! Like so many things in life, timing is everything.

The Problem with "But"

Saying "but" just doesn't work when you're trying to be validating. Imagine you're sitting down with your supervisor for your annual performance review.

"I just want you to know how much we all appreciate your hard work, your capacity to work independently, and your general good humor," she tells you. "You are liked by the people who report to you and valued by management, *but* there are a few things we need to look at."

Did you notice that everything before the *but* went out the window? Doesn't it seem like the really important stuff is going to come after the *but*? Somehow the earlier information, as important and accurate as it may be, is diminished just by the word *but*. Take a look at some more examples:

"I know you really loved him, *but* you will get over him."

"I can see how sad you are, *but* you will feel happy again."

"It makes sense that you're mad, *but* you can't carry on that way."

Both parts of these sentences can be true, *and* these statements probably wouldn't be experienced as validating. That's right—the magic word is *and*! If you're going to offer reassurance or problem solving in the same sentence—and I suggest that you avoid that as much as possible—please use *and* as the connector rather than *but*. Try substituting *and* for *but* in the examples above. Do you notice how the word *and* seems to make both ideas in the sentence of equal importance? Let the validation do its job before moving on to the next step.

Three Ways to Validate

Attentive listening, active listening, and giving voice to the unspoken are the three levels of validation that I want to teach you. Each of these skills builds on the previous one. I have no doubt that as you become more skillful with validation, you will be more helpful to your child. I would encourage you to start your validation practice at work or with friends. Get the hang of it in nonstressful situations outside the family, and then move to noncrisis situations within the family. If you practice developing the skill this way, you will be ready to use it when the emotional temperature is running high.

Sometimes it's difficult to determine whether you are being validating, so here's a clue. The easiest way to know is when the person tells you she feels understood. If she doesn't tell you directly, then notice whether she's telling you in more detail about the situation, especially if she's giving you more information about how she thinks or feels, rather than just details or facts. Does the person seem more relaxed and open compared to the beginning of the conversation? If so, then she probably felt validated.

Attentive Listening

Attentive listening is about posture, eye contact, and focus. With attentive listening, your entire attention is focused on the other person. It's as if nothing else in the universe is of any consequence—the only thing that matters is what the other person is saying. As you're listening, you're working at seeing the situation from his perspective. You need to pay attention to any judgments you're making. For example, are you telling yourself that he's wrong to feel the way he does, or that he's making too big a deal about his hurt or angry feelings? Judgments tend to distract us from truly being able to take another person's perspective. Notice these judgments and then let them go. Easier said than done, right? Especially when our emotionally vulnerable children seem poised on the precipice of a crisis that we think could be avoided if they could only gain some emotional perspective. In these moments our judgments often lead to comments that are invalidating. Here is an example of what I mean.

Mona's mother has been using her attentive listening skill for the last 10 minutes, but Mona is becoming increasingly distressed. Mom knows from past experiences that when Mona gets like this, she's liable to engage in self-harm. Judgments about Mona making too big a fuss over the matter enter Mom's mind.

"I hate myself! I wish I could disappear!" Mona complained.

"Oh, Mona! Don't you think that's a little over the top? After all, it wasn't that big a deal," Mother interjected.

"I can't believe you just said that. I thought you understood. I am done with this conversation!" Mona yelled as she fled to her bedroom.

So how do we let go of our judgments? The first step is to notice when judgments are arising in your mind. The second step is to accept that these judgments are likely to be counterproductive to your goal of validation. Then imagine that they are like clouds in the sky and let them pass. The key is not to let yourself get too attached to the "rightness" of your judgments. In fact, there may be a fair amount of "truth" in Mom's opinion that Mona's problem wasn't so important that she should hate herself, and for sure it wasn't worth dying over. Had Mona's mom been a bit better at managing her understandable worry and avoided her judgments, the interchange may have gone this way.

"I hate myself! I wish I could disappear!" Mona complained.

"Oh, Mona, you are really troubled by this. That's a terrible way to feel. Can I help?" Mona's mom asked.

"Not really. I'll get over it," Mona replied.

Of course, validation does not always work as smoothly as it did in this example, but it will give you a fighting chance to help your child lower her current emotional temperature. Lowered emotional temperature will help your child decide how to be more skillful to get through the crisis.

Active Listening

Attentive listening becomes active listening when we add the element of reflection or, as it's sometimes referred to, "mirroring." Reflection is simply restating the other person's feelings in the service of letting her know you follow her, or as a way to make sure you understand how she feels or thinks in the moment.

"I am feeling really down about Melissa moving to Dallas. We were just getting to be friends and now she's leaving," Joan said.

"I can see how down you are," Joan's dad replied.

When we are actively listening, we are not adding anything new to the discussion; we are simply trying to stay on point with the feelings being expressed. Some of the time it might not be altogether clear what emotion is being expressed, and active listening can help us both to clarify the emotion and to be validating at the same time.

"I am feeling really down about Melissa moving to Dallas. We were just getting to be friends and now she's leaving," Joan said.

"It sounds like you're sad about Melissa moving to Dallas," Joan's dad replied.

"Yeah, I am so bummed out."

In this example Joan's father uses active listening to get clear about what Joan means when she says she's "down." Staying open and curious about your child's experience are key factors in being successful at active listening. For some of us, when our worries or emotions begin to rise, we get locked into a sense of certainty about what's happening. Our thinking loses any flexibility; we can't be budged from our own point of view. We typically refer to such people as "stubborn."

"Mary did it again. I don't believe her. She is having a sleepover and she didn't invite me. I had to hear about it from Sheila. I could have died," Kate complained.

"It sounds like you are really mad at Mary," said Kate's dad.

"No, I'm not mad, I'm humiliated," Kate responded.

"I don't know—it seems like you're mad about it," Dad went on.

"Stop telling me what I feel! I hate when you do that," Kate said, the tension in her voice rising.

Kate's father gets stuck on what he thinks his daughter feels and will not give up his point of view. It would not be irrational for someone in Kate's position to feel mad at Mary—but that doesn't seem to be her experience. Kate's father's refusal to amend his position is most likely going to make the situation worse. When you're engaged in active listening as a

> *When you're engaged in active listening as a validation strategy, it's all about acknowledging the other person's experience as he or she is describing it. Think "mirror," not "mind reader."*

validation strategy, it's all about acknowledging the other person's experience as he or she is describing it. Think "mirror" and not "mind reader."

Another common problem with reflection is that it can come across as stilted or phony. This is very often the case when people are first learning the skill, so again my advice would be to practice the skill outside on neutral ground first. Finally, don't feel obligated to reflect every feeling as it arises in a conversation. Use your reflections just to let the other person know you're following him or her or as a way to help you get more clarity about his or her experience.

Giving Voice to the Unspoken

Giving voice to the unspoken is the most advanced category of validation that I'm going to teach you. I suggest waiting on this one until you feel confident that you have the hang of attentive listening and active listening. Giving voice to the unspoken requires you to be open, curious, and extremely focused on what the other person is expressing. Being open and curious requires that you let go of any judgments about how the other person should be feeling in the situation and just accept what she says. Being focused includes paying attention to her words as well as her facial expressions and body language. Paying attention to the nonverbal cues (body language and facial expressions) will lead you to giving voice to the unspoken.

Sometimes as you are listening to your child, you will notice that there is something she's telling you that goes beyond the words she's using. It could be that as she's telling you about how angry she is, you notice a look of sadness in her eyes; or as she tells you about something that embarrassed her, her posture takes on an angry quality. When you notice these unspoken feelings, you can give voice to them. Here is an example of what I mean.

"I'm furious with Lena. We were supposed to meet for lunch at the cafeteria and she just blew me off. I told her how important it was to me that we talk today. She just didn't show. Finally I tracked her down and she said Molly needed to talk with her about the trouble she was having with her boyfriend," Crystal said with a quiver in her voice. "She can be such an idiot."

Crystal's mother noticed the quiver in her daughter's voice and the cloud of sadness that seemed to move across her face.

"I certainly can understand how mad you are with Lena. But tell me, did her not showing up also hurt your feelings?" Crystal's mom inquired.

"Yeah, it hurt my feelings! I think I'm both mad and sad about the whole thing," Crystal replied.

See how Crystal's mom gave voice to feelings that her daughter had not yet articulated? Notice how she gently inquired, not from a position of certainty but from one of curiosity—unlike Kate's dad insisting that she seemed angry. It is very important that when using this validation skill, you don't become attached to the "correctness" of your point of view. If the other person doesn't confirm what you think she might have been feeling, *let it go*. If you don't, you are very likely to make the situation worse.

Often the wish to understand our children and to help them solve a problem makes us unwittingly committed to the belief that we understand a situation when we don't. Parents lose their curiosity, and misguided certainty takes its place. When we are using giving voice to the unspoken, we are quite vulnerable to committing this error. The trick is to stay aware of your mind shutting down. When you notice this occurring, reach for curiosity. Remain interested in understanding your child's experience without assuming that you already understand it. Here's another example.

Izzie had just returned from school and went directly to the kitchen. Today was the day she was going to hear if she made the varsity lacrosse team. Izzie is a sophomore and played J.V. last year with all her friends. She was the only sophomore who was being considered for varsity. All week she has worried about whether she was good enough and whether she wanted to leave her friends behind.

"Mom," she said. "I didn't make it."

"Well, I guess your worries are over. Now you'll be playing with your friends," her mom gently replied.

"Yeah, I guess you're right," Izzie said without much conviction.

"Gee, Izzie, all week long this has been such a worry for you, and now it's settled," her mom continued.

"I don't know why I am unhappy, but I am," Izzie said.

"I wonder if you aren't a little sad that you didn't make the team?" her mom asked.

"Yeah, that's it. I'm glad I'll be playing with my friends, but I also would have liked to have been chosen," she replied with relief in her voice.

Once again, notice that Mom remains curious and open to her daughter and that she offers another possibility with a light touch. Using a light touch with real curiosity is the key to this skill.

Getting more practiced at validation will, over time, help to avoid emotional turmoil at home. It will give you a better understanding of your child's emotional stresses and open up better lines of communication. I encourage you to practice validation every chance you have at work, with friends, and with family members. And don't forget to validate yourself for working hard at learning a new skill!

In this chapter I've given you some practical skills to help you help your child reset the stage to identify and work through her emotions. In the next chapter you'll learn a number of additional skills to help support your teen's acquisition of the emotion modulation skills that will make self-injury an unnecessary stopgap solution to emotional pain.

7

writing a better script
NEW WAYS TO DISCOURAGE SELF-INJURY

As valuable as validation is in helping your emotionally sensitive child, it's not a problem-solving strategy. This chapter focuses on skills you can learn—or polish—to help your teen develop emotion regulation skills and leave self-injury behind. After practicing and mastering these skills, you will, in a way, be rewriting the script of your child's emotional vulnerability to bring about a better outcome.

INTERPERSONAL EFFECTIVENESS SKILLS

In my experience parents and children often develop patterns or styles of relating that don't work well. When a parent is struggling to be helpful to a child who self-injures, these patterns often push the child into emotional dysregulation. In other cases parents can become so tentative in their requests or in setting limits that they seriously compromise their ability to parent. Watch what happens when Bonnie's mother hears some upsetting news.

"I'm going to see Kerri this Saturday night," Bonnie told her mom matter-of-factly.

"What! I can't believe I'm hearing this. Every time you and Kerri see each other you get into trouble. What are you thinking?" Bonnie's mom anxiously replied.

"That's not true! Besides, you can't tell me who I can see and who I can't," exclaimed Bonnie.

"This is a bad idea and you're not doing it," Mom firmly replied.

"F—— you!" Bonnie screamed as the front door slammed behind her.

I imagine that quite a few of you have been in a situation similar to this one. When tempers flare, there's no chance for either party to explain her thinking. The situation has been made much worse between Bonnie and her mother overall, and the issue about Saturday night remains unresolved. Let's take a look at another version of the conversation that doesn't work for a different reason.

"I'm going to see Kerri this Saturday night," Bonnie told her mom matter-of-factly.

"Oh, that's nice, I think. Umm, wasn't she the girl you had some trouble with? I don't know, do you think it's a good idea to see her?" Mom asked cautiously.

"What are you saying? When are you going to trust my judgment? I don't believe you!" Bonnie replied.

"It's not that I don't trust you, uh, it's just that I'm concerned," Bonnie's mom went on.

"This conversation is over! Maybe you ought to see a shrink about your crazy anxiety," Bonnie shouted as the door slammed behind her.

This time Bonnie's mom is walking on eggshells about her very real concerns. Her tentative approach backfires, and the conversation comes to a screeching halt.

The interpersonal effectiveness skills I'll review with you in this chapter are designed to help you avoid such tense and nonproductive interchanges. The skills are drawn directly from the interpersonal effectiveness module that your child learns in DBT and are divided into three groups:

- The skills required to ask for what you want or to say no to a request
- The skills required to repair or enhance a relationship
- The skills for setting a limit while holding on to your self-respect

In order to be interpersonally effective, the first thing you need to do is assess your goals or priorities for the conversation. A handy way to think about your goals is to ask yourself these questions:

- Am I making a request?
- Am I trying to set things right?
- Am I attempting to set a firm limit?

First, if you have more than one goal in a conversation, choose the most important one. Second, think of these skills as

> *Think of interpersonal effectiveness skills as dance steps. You may need to move fluidly between steps to get the dance right.*

dance steps, and of interpersonal effectiveness as a finely choreographed dance. You may need to move fluidly between steps (skill sets) to get the dance right.

Relationship Objective 1: Asking for What You Want or Saying No

When your top priority is to make a request or to say no, the mnemonic to re-member is DEAR MAN:

Describe
Express
Assert
Reinforce
(Stay) Mindful
Appear Confident
Negotiate

Here's how this skill breaks down. *Describe* is used to orient the other person to the situation you want to talk about. It's all about the facts. For ex-ample, "Last Saturday night you came in after curfew" or "On Tues-day you said you would clean your room." It's more useful to limit the discussion to one particular situation rather than speaking in generalities like "You always miss your curfew" or "I've asked you a thousand times to clean up your room." These kinds of state-ments usually put the other person on the defensive, which is not going to get you what you want.

> *Starting statements with "You" instead of "I" tends to put people on the defensive, which won't get you what you want from them.*

Next, *express* your feelings about the situation: "When you're late for curfew, I both worry about you and I get angry" or "When you say you're go-ing to clean your room and don't, I get really annoyed with you." Again, avoid general statements such as "You make me worry when you are late" or "You make me angry when you don't do what you say you're going to do." When you're expressing your feelings, it's important to remember to use state-ments that begin with "I" instead of "You." When you take responsibility for your feelings, your position in the conversation remains strong; when you at-tribute your feelings to the other person, you come across as simply reactive or as a victim.

Next in the sequence is to *assert* your request: "I want you to be home at the time we agreed upon" or "When you say you're going to clean your room at a certain time, I want you to do it." Your assertion needs to be clear and firm—no ifs, ands, or buts.

One of the best ways to reach your goal is to spell out what's in it for the person if she complies. This will *reinforce* your request. For example: "When you come in on time for your curfew, it makes it more likely that in the future I'd be willing to extend your time out" or "When you clean your room as you agreed you would, I won't have to nag you so much." When we find a way to reinforce behavior, we are increasing the probability of getting what we want. Whenever possible, the reinforcer should be a natural consequence of doing what you ask. For example, stay away from things like "If you come in on time, I'll get you the sweater you've been asking for" or "If you clean your room, you can have whatever you want for dinner." These certainly may get you what you want, but they're bribes that will work just for the moment, leaving you having to offer more and more in the future (and inviting rejoinders such as "Sure I'll come in on time, but what are you going to get me if I do?"). Stick to reinforcers that are a logical ("natural") outcome of meeting your request, like "When you come in on time that builds trust, and then I'll be more likely to extend your curfew in the future."

We all know how we can become distracted in these kinds of discussions. "Yeah, I know I was late for curfew, but what about all the times you're late picking me up from school? Do I make a fuss?" or "My room is a mess? Have you seen my sister's? Why don't you ever nag her about her room?" In the face of these often emotionally charged distractions, stay *mindful* of your objective. (I'll give you more help with developing mindfulness skills in Chapter 8, and you'll find sources of detailed information on mindfulness practices in the Resources at the back of the book.)

Remember, you are on a mission to reach your goal—don't get sidetracked. This means at times you are going to have to just plain ignore the distractions and repeat your request, and at other times you may have to defuse the situation. For example, "I would be happy to speak with you about arriving late to pick you up from school right after we finish the discussion about your curfew" or

> *You are on a mission to reach your goal—don't get sidetracked.*

"You might have a point about your sister's room. I'll listen to your opinion right after we get the issue about your room squared away." Mindfully giving your objective top priority will optimize the chances of realizing it.

It's also important that you *appear confident* when making your request. Notice I said "appear"—you can feel like Jell-O on the inside; you just have to look the part. Let's face it: sometimes it's really hard to make a request of your kid if you know it might lead to an emotionally charged scene. It makes sense that in the face of an anticipated fight, you may not feel as confident as you'd like to be. So play the part on the outside. How, you ask? Your posture should be upright but not rigid. Make good eye contact and keep your tone of voice even, almost matter-of-fact. I know this may seem a little hokey. If you think it's going to be difficult for you to look confident, try working at it in front of a mirror.

If it seems that you're not going to get exactly what you want and you're willing to be flexible, then—and only then—try to **negotiate**. Parents sometimes move to negotiation too quickly, depriving themselves of a greater chance of getting what they want. Be patient. But if you think the discussion is at a dead end, then you can move to negotiate.

DEAR MAN is a very useful and powerful skill. I suggest that you try writing it out and practicing it a few times before you actu-

> *Don't move to negotiation too quickly—you may be giving up a better shot at getting what you want.*

ally use it. When you're ready, try it out in relatively neutral situations with friends or at work before bringing it home. Let's see how Bonnie's mother rewrites her daughter's emotional script after she's practiced this skill for a while.

"I'm going to see Kerri this Saturday night," Bonnie told her mom matter-of-factly.

"When you announce what you're going to do, especially given the trouble you had last time you went out with Kerri, it raises my worry, and I am almost automatically going to say no. It would be better for me if you raised it as a question for us to discuss [describe and express, beginning of assert]," Bonnie's mom said calmly.

"Okay, what are you going to say if I raise it as a question?" Bonnie asked warily.

"I don't know. My decision would be based on the conversation we have. I can tell you that I'm much more likely to agree if I have a sense that you've taken my concerns seriously [reinforce]."

"What does this have to do with you? She's my friend, and I should decide who I spend my time with, not you," Bonnie said with some irritation.

"In part that's true. But right now we need to settle the issue of Saturday night [staying mindful of the objective and appearing confident]."

"Well, what do you want me to do? I want to see Kerri."

"I'd like Kerri to come here this time and see how it goes."

"No! We want to go to the mall."

"She can come here first, and if things go okay, I'll drop you off at the mall for an hour or so [negotiate]."

"I don't really like it, but I'll do it, I guess."

"Thank you." Bonnie's mom ends the conversation with a smile.

Relationship Objective 2: Repairing or Enhancing the Relationship

It is inevitable that we are going to do or say things that will hurt other people's feelings. It's just a fact of being in a relationship. Frequently the hurt occurs in the context of a heated interchange when both parties are under the sway of their emotions. In order for you to use this new skill effectively, you need to be calm and relatively sure that you'll be able to stay focused on your goal: repairing the relationship. Finding your way back to a calm state can be accomplished with the mindfulness practices and distress tolerance skills that will be outlined in Chapter 8. So wait on practicing this skill until you have read that chapter.

After you've read and practiced it, you can use the GIVE skill to make a repair. This skill can be very helpful to your child in ways that go beyond keeping your relationship on an even keel. After a blowup between parent and kid in a family where the emotional climate can run hot, often neither party mentions the fight. Things just settle back down to "normal" and everybody goes on as if nothing happened. Families get into this pattern as a way to avoid another troubling scene.

While the avoidance is understandable, there are at least four problems that are potentially generated by this pattern. First, there is little or no resolution about the issue that started the problem. Second, hurt feelings are not addressed, which, when left to linger, are going to start affecting the relationship over the long haul. Third, the kid has no effective model about how relationships are maintained. Parents who can model effective ways to repair relationships are teaching their kids an important life tool. All relationships, to one degree or another, require work, and one aspect of that work is knowing how to make a repair when things go sour. Fourth, one of the tasks of adolescence, one that is especially difficult for emotionally vulnerable children, is the construction of a sense of time. I will address this issue in more detail at the end of the chapter, but here is the short version.

Emotionally vulnerable adolescents sometimes seem to have a snapshot view of time. Often the emotional fight you and she had in the morning, which practically ruined your day, appears to be disconnected from whatever she is asking from you in the afternoon—as if the fight no longer has any relevance. These kids have an exaggerated sense of "That was then and this is now" syndrome. They don't experience life so much as an ongoing series of events that are connected, like in a movie, as like a scrapbook full of still pictures. This snapshot view of the world is only confirmed when conflicts don't get addressed in an ongoing way.

Emotionally vulnerable kids often have a "snapshot" rather than a "movie" view of events. Do your best to give them more of a continuous "movie" view of their lives.

It's important that parents work at modeling the movie version of life, and one way to do that is through relationship repair. And one way to do *that* is with the GIVE skill:

(Be) Gentle
(Act) Interested
Validate
Easy manner

It almost goes without saying that if your objective is to repair a relationship, your demeanor needs to be **gentle**. Being gentle includes a soft tone of voice, being nondefensive, and being open to examining your contribution to the problem. This is why my advice to you was not to initiate the **give** skill until you're sure you'll be able to be gentle. Take whatever time you need, and do some mindfulness exercises or use some of the crisis survival strategies from the distress tolerance module (Chapter 8) to get ready. Once you're able to be gentle, the next step is to bring a degree of **interest** in hearing the other person's point of view. You want to convey your interest in whatever point of view your kid was articulating before the conversation went south.

Notice how, in the following exchange, Jackie seems to compartmentalize what happened in the morning as somewhat disconnected from the present. It doesn't have the same relevance for her as it does for her father. The simple act of tying the morning to the present helps to undercut her snapshot view of time.

"Jackie, I'm sorry that we had words this morning. I know you felt hurt and angry by my remarks. Do you think we could try again?" Jackie's dad gently inquired.

"I don't want to talk about it! It's over, done—that was this morning, this is now. Leave me alone. Anyway if we talk you'll just get mad at me again," Jackie said.

"Hey, give me a second chance. I know I was unreasonable this morning. I have a hard time thinking clearly when your music is so loud, and I didn't do such a good job of trying to talk to you about it," Dad replied.

"Okay. But remember, the music I listen to is important to me. When you tell me it's 'crap,' I really get upset," said Jackie.

Jackie's father doesn't have to be interested in his daughter's music one iota. He does, however, have to *act* interested to make sure the repair is effective. If you can't act interested in the thing that tipped over the conversation, then get interested in why the issue is so important to your child. Acting interested is accomplished by making good eye contact, carefully following the thread of the conversation, being curious, and asking relevant questions. Acting interested will help you be more effective at the third component of the skill, **validation**.

By now you are all experts at validation, so I'm not going to repeat the how-tos of this skill. Let's move on to the last component of GIVE, using an *easy manner*.

Back to Jackie and her dad.

"Okay. But remember, the music I listen to is important to me. When you tell me it's 'crap,' I really get upset," Jackie said.

"I can see how that would make you angry and hurt your feelings. Hey, but maybe you could cut me some slack—I never grew out of the Beatles," Jackie's dad replied.

Using an *easy manner* requires that we find a way to bring a light touch to the discussion. We want to ramp down the intensity and stay matter of fact. A little bit of humor can go a long way to helping create an easy manner. If you're going to use humor, I would suggest that it be more self-deprecating than teasing of the other person. Remember: your goal is repair, and you don't want to risk offending the other person.

Relationship Objective 3: Setting a Limit and Holding on to Your Self-Respect

It's a tough job, but someone's got to do it. Part of parenting is being able to set limits. Parents of an emotionally vulnerable child who engages in self-injury have an even tougher job because setting effective limits increases the likelihood of making the child emotionally dysregulated. If they don't set limits, they're dodging one set of problems for a whole host of others. The bottom line is that all kids need limits, and emotionally vulnerable kids particularly benefit from them.

Often an emotionally vulnerable child is triggered by too much discussion about an issue that is not negotiable. The endless discussion just serves to increase the child's emotional volatility. Some parents know they should be setting a limit, but avoid it and then feel guilty that they have abdicated a responsibility. Over time the guilt begins to erode a parent's sense of self-respect. Other parents go in the opposite direction and set limits like gangbusters, overreacting and being too harsh. Coming on too strong is sometimes born from frustration, or it can be a way to make sure they don't avoid the responsibility. In either case, feelings are hurt on all sides and parental self-respect is a casualty.

Effective limit setting is a skill you can learn, but of all the interpersonal effectiveness strategies, it may be the hardest to implement. If you've been the kind of parent who has avoided setting limits, things are probably going to have to get worse before they get better, as they did for Ruth.

"I understand that it's important for you to see your boyfriend on Saturday night, but I will not allow you to be at his house alone," Ruth firmly told her daughter Sarah.

"What? Come on. Have you gone crazy? It never mattered to you before," Sarah shot back.

"It did matter to me, but I was afraid I would upset you if I said no," Ruth confessed.

"Well, that's not my problem. It just isn't fair—you just can't change the rules like that!" Sarah complained.

"I can see how it might seem unfair, but the answer is still no," Ruth replied.

"I'm not going to follow your stupid rules!" Sarah wailed as she slammed the door.

Ruth may be in for several more go-rounds before Sarah begins to settle in to the new way of doing things. If, however, Ruth is unable to hold her course and gives in to Sarah, she will reinforce her daughter's argumentativeness. I'm not suggesting that you be rigid and inflexible with your limits; *just don't change them in the face of your kid's dysfunctional behavior.* Renegotiate limits when your child is in emotional control and has made a convincing case for change.

The skill for effective limit setting is FAST:

(Be) Fair
(No) Apologies
Stick to your values
(Be) Truthful

You want to be *fair* to yourself and the other person. Notice how Ruth validates both her daughter's wish to see her boyfriend and the fact that changing the rules has an element of unfairness to it. When you're being fair, you are undercutting any tendency to blame the other person—and when blame is out of the equation, limit setting goes more smoothly.

No *apologies* really means no excessive apologizing. When you're setting a limit, it works best if you're direct and somewhat matter of fact. Avoid statements like "I'm really sorry to have to ground you. I wish I didn't have to do this." These kinds of apologies undercut your goal and open the door to fruitless discussion. Any teenager worth her salt is either going to tell you that you don't have to be burdened by guilt, just don't set the limit, or she's going to accuse you angrily of not being sorry at all. Just don't go down that path.

We often set limits when a particular value of ours has been crossed or is about to be. Ruth's value is that it's not okay. to be at a boy's house without adult supervision. Sticking **to your values** requires you to be clear about what's important and nonnegotiable versus those issues where you may have some flexibility to negotiate. Sometimes parents or caretakers have different values from each other, and sometimes those differing values become apparent only when one parent is either setting a limit or expecting the partner to do so. When this occurs it's important that the adults involved discuss their differing points of view and decide on a course of action.

Often parents feel the need to have these discussions privately, which is a perfectly reasonable way to go. But there's often some benefit for parents in clarifying their differing sets of values and deciding on a course of action in front of the child. Having the discussion in private deprives our kids of seeing how conflict is reasonably resolved. Of course, if you think the discussion is going to get heated and contentious, then taking it behind closed doors is the way to go.

When we set limits, it's important to remain **truthful**. Notice how open Sarah's mom is about her past behavior of letting her daughter be at the boy-

> *If you and your partner disagree on values or limit setting, it's sometimes useful to hash it out in front of your child. This will teach him or her how conflicts can be resolved reasonably. But don't stage a heated confrontation in front of your child.*

friend's house alone. I'm sometimes amazed at the creativity that parents harness in the service of preventing their child from doing something while avoiding the truth. (No Sarah, it is not that we don't trust you to be alone, it's just that we want you to spend the night with old Aunt Jennie.) If you're avoiding the truth as a way of dodging an argument, you're settling for a short-term solution to a longer term problem. Setting limits helps children learn how to manage disappointment, and wouldn't you agree that learning how to make it through disappointing times is an important life skill?

Being truthful is not the same as being brutally honest, so by all means deliver a truthful message in a sensitive manner. Your goal is to set a limit, and the degree to which you can do that without being hurtful will aid you in accomplishing that goal.

INDIRECT INTERPERSONAL SKILLS

Validation and interpersonal effectiveness are skills that you can actively and directly use to be helpful to your child. There are other changes you can make in the way you parent that are less direct but will also be helpful in steering your teenager away from self-harming behaviors. Demonstrating your capacity to manage distressing events and the ways you cope with the difficult emotions that accompany these events is important modeling for your kid. This kind of modeling has the potential to help your child get better at effectively managing these painful moments in his own life.

In addition, all kids need the sense of security that comes with having parents who pay attention to them but who also know when to give them some privacy. Effectively and flexibly responding to these two issues helps the child feel understood while giving him a sense that you will extend trust to him when he is managing his emotions more effectively.

Often when we try to protect our children from the natural consequences of their behavior, we unwittingly communicate our sense that they are handicapped or damaged in some way. So knowing when to allow natural consequences to unfold will help your child develop a more resilient sense of himself. The changes that I will outline are about creating an environment that will support and enhance validation, interpersonal effectiveness, and your child's individual therapy. Probably the single most effective action that you can take to help your kid is to make sure he's in effective treatment. Once that's accomplished, here are some other strategies that will be of help.

Modeling Distress Tolerance

One of the most powerful ways that kids learn skills is by watching the adults around them. When we employ skillful behavior we are not only helping ourselves; we are modeling effective behavior for our children to learn. As you know, one of the central difficulties for the vast majority of children who engage in self-harming behavior is not being able to modulate and tolerate painful emotions. When under the sway of these powerful and uncomfortable emotions, these children are in a rush to change the way they feel. They lack the capacity to sit with their internal discomfort and are prone to move quickly into action. When parents sense that their child is in distress, they often unwittingly join them in the rush to change the situation. This is what happens to Tameka and her mom.

> *Under the sway of powerful and uncomfortable emotions, these children are in a rush to change the way they feel.*

"I need to speak to Jimmie right now! He's not picking up his cell phone. I have to know what's going on with us. I can't take not knowing," Tameka complained.

"Have you tried his land line?" Tameka's mom asked, sensing her daughter's distress.

"Of course! I'm not stupid," Tameka angrily replied.

"Try his cousin—you know he hangs out there all the time," Mom said as her anxiety began to rise. "It worries me to see you so upset."

"I hate his cousin. You know that! Leave me alone," Tameka shouted.

Tameka's mom moves right to problem solving. In her own hurry to help her child, she joins her in her frantic need to get things resolved immediately. Tameka's mother skips validation and begins to offer unsolicited advice—and gets the predictable negative result. In the second example, Tameka's mom takes a longer view, modeling the capacity to tolerate distress.

"I need to speak to Jimmie right now! He's not picking up his cell phone. I have to know what's going on with us. I can't take not knowing," Tameka complained.

"It's so hard to wait, especially about your relationship with Jimmie," Tameka's mom replied.

"I'm going to jump out of my skin. Why doesn't he answer my calls?" Tameka responded with sadness in her voice.

"I'm sorry that he hasn't returned your calls. Waiting is really hard. I tell you what, why don't we bake some cookies while you wait? Maybe that will make the time pass by faster," offered Tameka's mother.

"That's not going to help! I can't stand this!" Tameka shouted.

"You're right—it's not going to get Jimmie to call you any sooner, but it just may make waiting easier," said her mother.

"I guess you're right about that. Do we have any chocolate chips?" asked Tameka.

This time Tameka's mom does several things differently. First, she takes the time to validate her daughter's experience by acknowledging how difficult waiting can be. Second, she does not offer any problem-solving strategies, but models distress tolerance. She does this when she acknowledges that making cookies is not going to solve the problem but may ease some of the distress caused by the waiting. And third, she does not seem to be getting caught up in her daughter's increasing emotional temperature. This is a hard-won parental skill. Mom seems to have accepted the situation as it is, and is now just offering a way to manage a problem that can't be solved right now. By exhibiting these distress tolerance skills, she's showing Tameka how to do the same.

Obviously, it's not easy to model distress tolerance if you, like your teenager, are relatively sensitive emotionally and you haven't fully developed emotion modulation skills. Chapter 8 will help you build your own skills further so you can help yourself and your teen.

Privacy Versus Increased Vigilance

One of the most challenging problems for parents with kids who engage in self-harm is knowing when to allow them privacy and when to become more vigilant. Unfortunately, there aren't any hard-and-fast rules about this. There are only some guidelines or principles to help you think this through. Whatever course of action you take, however, make sure your child understands what to expect and knows that her therapist has been informed of your decisions.

The first thing to hold in your mind is that there are few if any interventions that anyone can make to prevent someone from self-injuring. Your more modest goal is to make your child feel noticed and understood when she's in crisis through the use of validation, and to give her more privacy when you see that she's more skillfully managing her emotions. Ask her how she's feeling, gently inquire about what's on her mind and how she's doing—I will refer to this as "checking in." Here are some examples of how this principle gets translated into everyday life.

First, let your child know, in moments of relative calm, that when she's in emotional turmoil, you expect her to let you in on it. Let her know very clearly that if she wants your help, it's there for the asking; if she doesn't, you expect her to use some technique or skill to help herself. Second, when she's having trouble she should expect you to be checking in with her more frequently than usual. What you want your child to know is that the objective in checking in is to see how she's doing and whether she wants any help from you. Your intention is not to bug her but only to be supportive.

Don't expect your child to welcome your increased vigilance. She may

> *Learn to check in with your child lightly: just gently ask her how she's doing.*

even tell you that it won't prevent her from self-injuring or that it will only make the situation worse. My advice is to gently stick to your guns and let her know that she's correct—it won't prevent her from self-harming. Furthermore, if checking in really becomes a problem, you need to be willing to review the strategy down the line. If, over time, you feel it's doing more harm than good, then discard this strategy and concentrate on the others outlined in this chapter.

When you are checking in, use a light touch, practice validation, and stay away from problem solving unless invited to do so. If your kid says everything is fine and you clearly see that it isn't, let it go and just keep checking in.

How often should you check in with your child? That's something you'll have to figure out by trial and error. It will also depend on how troubled your kid is in the moment and, to some degree, how smoothly the check-ins are going. If you think your child is in better emotional control, then decrease the frequency of checking in. You'll just have to feel your way through this process.

Allowing Natural Consequences

As parents we have an instinctual inclination to protect our children from hardships. There are times, however, when this inclination can have a detrimental effect. In these moments we may be reinforcing the kid's sense that she is so weak or damaged that she has to be protected from the natural consequences of her behavior. We may be inadvertently sending the message that she can't emotionally handle the problem, rather then helping her tolerate the distress that accompanies the problem. Watch what happens with Jody's parents.

"Jody's school called today," Jody's mom told Jody's father. "One of the kids in her class noticed the cuts on her arm and told the guidance counselor. The guidance counselor called the nurse, who called me and left a message on the answering machine. She wants to know if we think there's a problem. What should we do?"

"There's no way I want the school to know that she cut herself again! If they find out, Jody won't be able to play lacrosse this spring. You know they get rigid about this kind of stuff. Jody's been miserable enough—she doesn't need more stress," Jody's dad replied.

"What are we going to do? I don't feel comfortable lying about what's going on. After all, the school has been pretty supportive so far. I don't want to screw things up with them," Jody's mom responded.

What would you do if you had to wrestle with this dilemma? Jody's dad's position seems entirely reasonable; he wants to protect his daughter and minimize the stress in her life. On the other hand, his wife's worry that lying to the school could potentially backfire is also reasonable. The central question is how to make the best guess about what's in Jody's best interest. One way to tackle this problem is to make a Pros and Cons Chart about the various options. Actually, you need two Pros and Cons Charts, the first one assessing the short-term consequences of the decision and the second the longer term consequences. Doing pros and cons is a pretty standard method for thinking through complex decisions. It's especially useful in situations where rational thinking is paramount, but emotions are liable to run high and compromise the process. The structured nature of doing pros and cons can guard against emotions taking the day. At times you may want to have your child be part of this exercise. If he's been in a DBT treatment, he has most likely learned this skill already.

For the situation with Jody, the Pros and Cons Chart that will yield the most thorough information would look like this:

Short-Term Consequences

Pros	Cons
Telling the school: maintain good relations with the school	No lacrosse
Not telling the school: maintain Jody's privacy	Deprive Jody of school support

Spend some time with your own ideas about Jody's parents' dilemma. Add to this chart, and create one for the long-term consequences. Here are some ideas for starting points. One long-term consequence under the pros category about telling the school is that Jody will experience the natural consequences of her actions. The school may decide that from its perspective, she needs a limited schedule that would eliminate lacrosse. Feeling the pinch of this loss may help Jody become more committed to using her therapy to end self-injurious behavior. A con of Jody's parent's withholding information from the school is that it might move Jody's thinking in the direction that self-injury is not so much of a problem if she can keep it secret.

As you can see, there are any number of legitimate ways to think about whether to intervene in your child's life or to allow natural consequences to occur. There is no one right answer, just some effective routes to help you make your decisions.

I know there may be a lot of new information in this chapter, so take your time, become familiar with the strategies, and pay attention to the small successes. You can't help your child if you put too much pressure on yourself or your child to change quickly. When you're taking care of yourself, you will have the energy and the resilience to parent your child. The next chapter focuses more specifically on how you can take care of the pain and distress that comes with having a child who is struggling.

8

taking care of yourself
to take care of your teen

I don't have to tell you that parenting a child who engages in self-injury is extremely hard work. The stress and anxiety take a toll, and you may feel exhausted, defeated, and hopeless. Parental burnout is a debilitating experience. Some common indicators of burnout include sleep problems, changes in appetite, general irritability, depressed mood, and increased alcohol consumption. Your self-esteem can take a nosedive, leading you to question every parenting move you ever made. You can lose perspective on your parenting abilities. Guilt and remorse can become your constant companions. Some parents withdraw from their children's problems and become over involved in work or other kinds of activities in an effort to avoid their feelings of helplessness and pain. Others become overly focused on their child's difficulties at the expense of a life outside the home.

SIGNS AND SYMPTOMS OF PARENTAL BURNOUT

1. Increased difficulties in significant relationships.
2. Increased irritability and/or lack of patience.
3. Significant decrease in pleasurable activities.
4. Increased alcohol use.
5. Changes in appetite.
6. Sleep difficulties.
7. Increased sense of loneliness and isolation.
8. Persistent anxiety and rumination.

SIBLINGS

In some families the child who is self-harming becomes too much of the focus; brothers or sisters can feel neglected. Often they don't protest or talk about how the lack of attention is affecting them because they're sensitive to their parents' worry. Their silence often misleads parents into thinking they're just fine. It's not unusual for some siblings to become anxious or withdrawn. Others make their protest known by their own behavior problems or academic difficulties.

It's extremely challenging and at times draining for parents to stay focused on the other children in the family, helping them understand what's going on while taking care of the sibling who self-injures: negotiating the mental health system, dealing with the school, and managing extended family. I will address these complex and difficult issues in the next chapter. This chapter is all about strategies to keep yourself on an even keel in the midst of a gale.

PARTNERS

A second casualty of burnout can be you and your partner. Whether you're married, living with your partner, or living separately, your capacity to be effective in relationships goes out the window when you're suffering from burnout. Relationships take care and attention. When we're fatigued in mind, body, and spirit, that can seem to take more energy than we have in the tank. If you notice that you have significantly less patience and understanding for the other person, or feel that the other person is being intentionally mean, or have the feeling that your side of the story is not being heard and valued, then you probably need to examine the relationship. As difficult as it sometimes is to maintain a relationship, it will pay off in helping you avoid parental burnout.

DIVORCED PARENTS

Divorced parents who have worked well together in the past often find that the new challenges presented by a child who is self-injuring require adjustments. Furthermore, the need for increased communication between divorced couples can put a strain on whatever new love interests the parents may be developing.

If, however, what I have described has gone on between you and your parenting partner for years but just gets worse in stressful situations, then it's probably not burnout. It may be that you and your partner have a conflict that you've been unable to resolve. Often problems in parenting, when you follow them back to the core, are really problems in the relationship between the parents. Solutions can be as simple as learning to communicate better or as complicated as addressing a past betrayal. Whatever its source, it is most definitely a problem that needs to be addressed.

Chronic parenting problems are always a challenge, but when a child is having serious emotional trouble, it is imperative that couples find a way to work at making improvements in their relationship. Couple therapy, therapy focused on guiding parents, and/or individual counseling may help you resolve these issues. If, however, you've tried to work things out and where you are with your partner is as good as it gets, then it's especially important that you use other strategies to take care of yourself.

SINGLE PARENTS

Single parents have a unique set of challenges. Often the support network of family and friends you may have relied on in the past is not a viable resource anymore. That may be due to your reluctance to reach out to them because of feelings of shame and guilt, or because you don't feel your network of people would be supportive of your child who self-harms. If that's the case, you can feel extremely lonely and isolated, even trapped or resentful of your parenting role. All parents are susceptible to doubt, self-blame, and remorse, but the single parent is particularly vulnerable to these draining experiences.

For all kinds of parents of children who self-injure, learning how to take care of yourself and the parenting relationship may take the edge off the difficult times ahead. What can you do to keep burnout at bay, or at least diminish its effects? In the following sections I will teach you some skills to helping you avoid feeling overwhelmed by negative emotions. These skills are all part of the emotion regulation and distress tolerance modules from the DBT skills curriculum. You will recognize them from my review of teens' work in DBT from Part I. Once you start taking better care of yourself, you'll have more energy and resilience to hang in there through the rough times with your child.

ACCEPTANCE VERSUS PROTEST, RESIGNATION, AND DESPAIR

"Sometimes I can't believe this is happening!" Kris's mother said with a tinge of anger in her voice. "Kris never had any problems before. I thought she was doing so well—then she made these new friends, and the next thing we know, she's cutting herself. It seems that nothing her dad and I do makes a difference. Some days I don't even want to get out of bed."

I'm sure many of you can identify with Kris's mother. At times it may seem that feeling resigned, angry, and hopeless is all you can expect. While it's natural to experience these emotions, they needn't take over your life. In fact, remaining in such a state will only lead to more exhaustion and a more depressed mood—increasing the probability of burnout.

Fortunately there is a way out. Here are some practical steps that are most likely to lead you to a better emotional place. Remember that learning new skills takes patience, practice, and perseverance.

Step 1: Becoming Mindfully Aware of the Way Things Are

Slow yourself down by paying attention to your breathing. You don't have to breathe any special way; just focus your attention on your breath. When you are a bit more centered, turn your attention to your current emotions, thoughts, and sensations. Take a moment and just notice what you are thinking and feeling and the accompanying bodily sensations. You may find that you have some judgments about your thoughts and feelings—just notice them and let them pass. For example, you may notice your thought that a stronger or more resilient person wouldn't feel the way you do or that it isn't fair that this is happening to you. Let it go. I guarantee you these judgments are not useful to you.

If you find that you have some trouble letting the judgments pass, here are some techniques to try. Imagine that your judgments are like clouds in the sky and just watch them float away. Or picture yourself putting the judgments on a conveyor belt and watching them disappear from view.

The first step is just about noticing how things are—period.

Step 2: Letting Go

Once you have noticed what you're feeling, thinking, or sensing, the next order of business is about accepting the situation as it is. Nonacceptance reflects itself through tension in our bodies, repetitive thoughts about not believing the situation we are in is occurring, and feeling angry and/or sad.

Here's what you need to do. Slow your breathing down and notice where in your body you are holding the tension. Often we hold tension in the face or upper back, but learn where you yourself typically hold on to tension. Then deliberately relax that area of your body. Think about softening the muscles, or imagine the area getting warm and relaxed. Gently and kindly begin to tell yourself that things are as they are. Remind yourself that everything changes, and the current situation will pass. Stick with this process until you feel some relief.

Acceptance can be hard to come by, as we tend to use our imaginations to construct alternative scenarios. We can say to ourselves, "If only such-and-such hadn't happened, then I wouldn't be in the unfortunate place I find myself." Using our imaginations this way is bound to compound our misery. It makes us focus on what could or should have been. When that occurs we're likely to distract ourselves with an internal narrative that, while it could have been true, just doesn't match what's happening in real life. Or we can become immersed in creating a story about the future that leads us astray from effectively managing what is on our plates right now.

Acceptance is about acknowledging what's happening in the moment—whether it's planning your child's treatment, having a terrible argument with your spouse, or enjoying your dinner. Acceptance does not mean that you like what is happening or that you're in agreement with it, only that the facts are what the facts are. Remember when Kris's mom said she couldn't believe what was happening? That statement indicates that she has not yet fully accepted her situation (see box). When you accept things as they are, you'll often feel a sense of relief or calmness. Not accepting your situation is a direct route to increased suffering.

EXAMPLES OF PHRASES THAT INDICATE LACK OF ACCEPTANCE

1. This can't be happening.
2. This just isn't fair.
3. Why does this always happen to me/us/her?
4. I just will not deal with this.

Not long ago during a session in which we were teaching acceptance skills to parents of kids in our program, a mother reported the following experience. She told the group that while she knew that her kid was having troubles, she'd never really accepted this fact. She went on to say that she realized that she spent inordinate amounts of time thinking that this couldn't be really happening to her, that it was just a phase her child was going through. She even had the idea that she would wake up one morning to find that it had all been a dream. She told us she was in a constant state of worry and fear.

During the week after this session, she practiced acceptance and noticed the following: her anxiety decreased, she felt more able to harness her energies to help her child, she was sleeping better, and she was more effective at work. You have no doubt used acceptance skills in other parts of your lives without realizing it. Think about a time when you were stuck in traffic, or when you got some bad news at work, or you heard that your favorite sports team lost. You found a way to accept these situations and felt that you had a little more inner peace. The idea is to bring that same skill set to the current situation you are facing with your child.

Pain, as we know all too well, is an inevitable part of life. There's no way to avoid all of life's painful situations: people die, people get sick, and decisions we make turn out badly. Suffering, however, is another matter. Often we suffer because we won't accept the pain in our lives; we rail against the injustice of it all. The Buddhist tradition has an equation that says

Pain + Nonacceptance = Suffering

Acceptance occurs when we're no longer fighting reality but acknowledging our situation as it is in this moment. Acceptance helps to ease the inner emotional turmoil that is produced when we fight reality. That inner fight is one of the chief contributors to a sense of despair, impotent anger, and mental exhaustion that only leads to increased suffering.

Step 3: Repeating Steps 1 and 2

It turns out that acceptance can evaporate faster than dew on a summer morning. All too frequently our minds make a U-turn and we head right back toward rumination and suffering. The trick is to hold in your mind that acceptance doesn't often keep for long and you are very willing to start the process all over again. Acceptance can bring relief as long as we remain committed to working at it.

I first encountered the idea of acceptance as a strategy to help manage distress in my first formal DBT training. Soon after returning to Boston from the training, I found myself stuck in traffic that was going to make me very late for an important meeting. Naturally I'd left my cell phone at home. I began to do what I frequently did in such moments: I castigated myself for being so dumb as to leave the cell phone at home, I thought about how unjust it was that traffic was snarled when I was in a hurry, and I lathered myself into a near rage. Then I had the idea that maybe this was a time to practice acceptance.

"Okay," I said to myself. "First focus on your breath, then notice where the tension is in your body." I relaxed the muscles in my face and back. "Okay, now accept the situation as it is. You are stuck in traffic and you are going to be late. This is just how it is in this moment. Whatever is going to happen is going to happen, and there is currently nothing you can do to change the situation." Relief! Then, approximately 3 seconds later, "Crap! I'm stuck in traffic! This acceptance stuff is nonsense!" I shouted out loud. That's when I remembered to repeat steps 1 and 2.

Acceptance is not a problem-solving strategy, although it's often the first step in effective problem solving. If you think about it, you really can't find solutions to problems until you have accepted your circumstances as they are. Here is an example that I think will illuminate this point.

One day you go to your garage to start your car. You get in and turn on the ignition and you hear that whiny "no way is it going to start" sound. What do you do? If you're like most people, you turn the key several more times, as if that will make a difference. You now have a choice: you can complain about how this should not be happening and worry that you might have to buy a new car, all the while turning the key again and again, or you can accept things as they are and call AAA. Remember: acceptance does not require you to find your situation a good one; it just means acknowledging what's happening in this moment.

> *You can't find solutions to problems until you have accepted your circumstances as they are.*

EMOTIONAL MINDFULNESS

"You're going to do what? There's no way your mom and I are going to let you spend the night at Julia's house," Morgan's father shouted.

"Why not?" Morgan asked, her voice beginning to rise in anger.

"The very fact that you have to ask blows my mind," her father replied angrily. "Don't you remember what happened last time? You and she drank in her basement, had boys over late at night, and got involved in things that triggered your cutting."

"That won't happen again. I don't have any money for beer. Remember, you stopped my allowance!" Morgan shouted.

"That's not the point! You really can't be that dumb. When are you go-ing to grow up?" Morgan's father screamed.

Most parents I know—whether they're part of my clinical practice, friends, or relatives—have had the experience of becoming emotionally over-whelmed with anger and frustration in the face of some seemingly outlandish aspect of their teenager's behavior. They often report that in spite of their best intentions or efforts, they lose their emotional balance and fan the flames of the heated discussion. Often in the midst of the emotional storm the parents have the idea that their own reactions are making the situation worse, yet feel helpless in the moment to stop. That inner voice says, "Slow down—you're losing it," but they just can't harness sufficient restraint. Soon afterward, they feel guilt and remorse.

Sound familiar? It's a lousy feeling. Parents who have an emotionally vulnerable adolescent and one who is engaged in deliberate self-harm fre-quently worry whether their loss of emotional balance is going to trigger an act of self-injury. Some parents tell me that the most painful and crazy aspect of this moment is that sometimes, alongside the worry about causing their child to self-injure, is the goading thought, "Okay, kid, if you're going to hurt yourself, go ahead and do it," followed immediately by shame, guilt, and re-morse.

The overwhelming majority of parents I have met are extremely trou-bled by these kinds of experiences and struggle with the very painful feelings that linger for some time after the event. Knowing how to sidestep these situ-ations will help you feel better about yourself, guaranteed. So here is a tech-nique that can keep you from being swept away by your own emotional tidal wave: become mindfully aware of your feelings *before* they escalate to a trou-blesome point. Here is an example of what I mean.

Your daughter has been on the phone fighting with her boyfriend for the last half hour. Suddenly you hear the door to the bathroom slam shut. With-out even thinking, you rush upstairs and pound on the door, telling her to open up right now. She shouts back, telling you to leave her alone, that she's fine. You persist, which only leads to a heated exchange.

If you'd been able to be mindful of your emotions, the situation might have played out differently. You would have noticed that you were frightened of what your daughter was going to do, and for good reason, but noticing your fear might have slowed you down and enabled you to be more effective. In-stead of pounding on the door, you might have knocked, asked your daughter if she was okay, and communicated your worry. This might have avoided the fight.

When we can identify and accurately label our emotions, we are build-ing a kind of mental box that helps keep them safely contained, and we are

avoiding that awful sense of being
ambushed by our own emotions. Of
course, the situation is made more
complex when we're experiencing
more than one emotion at a time,
but our task is the same.

Say your child has been in
DBT therapy for about 6 weeks and
has been doing really well. After she

> *When we can identify and
> accurately label our emotions, we
> are building a kind of mental box
> to contain them safely—plus we
> avoid that awful sense of being
> ambushed by our own emotions.*

gets a bad grade on a math test, however, you notice some new scratches on
her arm. Almost without thinking, with annoyance in your voice, you confront her. The situation quickly deteriorates into an argument. If you'd been
able to be more mindful of your emotions, you might have noticed that while
you were angry, your stronger emotions were fear and sadness. Being more at-
tuned to all the emotions would most likely have helped you avoid the argument.

When we're successful in this process, we're less likely to be pulled into
the undertow of an emotional high tide. When our emotions just take us
over, in the language of DBT, we are in "emotion mind." In this state our
thoughts and actions are governed primarily by our powerful emotional experience; we have the feeling of being pushed around by our emotions. To the
degree that we're even thinking rationally, it seems to have no effect on our
actions.

From a neurobiological perspective, the parts of the brain that fire our
emotions are going full blast, while the parts of the brain that have to do with
rational thinking and problem solving have shut down. The trick is to get the
brain systems of the prefrontal cortex, which are responsible for rational
thought and action, back on line.

One way to do this is use the DBT skill called "mindfulness of your current emotion." As with any new skill, practice this one in situations of relative calm before employing it in the heat of an emotional firestorm. Practice
it when you miss the bus, when your favorite sports team loses, or when that
new recipe you spent all afternoon on makes an inedible mess. The two hypo-
thetical examples I just described with your child are typical situations where
this skill can really make a difference.

Step 1: Turning Your Attention to the Experience of the Emotion

Once again, the first step is to focus on the sensations that accompany the
emotion. Try to locate where in your body you feel the emotion. Your job is to
become a kind of anthropologist who is gently interested and curious to un-

derstand all aspects of a particular behavior. For example, most people when they are sad feel heaviness in their chest; they may also experience a tightening in their face as a way to prevent the tears from flowing and a trembling in their lips. When we're angry, we feel a tightening of our fists as our jaws move forward. Notice how the intensity of the feeling waxes and wanes.

The trick is to begin observing and describing these sensations as soon as you become aware that you're getting emotionally charged up. Your task is to simply notice what you're feeling; that's it. Doing this simple exercise will decrease the chances of things escalating into an altercation. Notice whether you're making any judgments about your emotions ("I am wrong to feel angry" or "It's dumb to feel sad") and, if you are, work at letting the judgments go. In a nonjudgmental fashion, just accept this moment as it is. By deliberately observing and describing your experience, you will bring your prefrontal cortex into play. When that happens, you'll find that you're more likely to become more rational and balanced.

For example, Ariel's mom noticed new cuts on her daughter's legs. Her first impulse was to ask her daughter what the heck was going on. Instead she noticed that she felt anger rising in her chest and some sadness alongside it. As she did this, she was able to put things in perspective and think about how she was going to address her observations with her daughter. What was surely headed toward a heated exchange now had a chance to become a controlled discussion.

Step 2: Doing What the Situation Requires

It may be that as you feel in more control you'll want to continue the discussion, or it may be that you need a break and will come back to the issue at a later time. Sometimes after regaining emotional control, what you need is to do something kind and soothing for yourself. Karen realized in the middle of confronting her daughter about her self-injury that she no longer felt tongue-tied by frustration and could calmly talk about it with her daughter. Sidney felt such an overwhelmingly heavy sadness when his son explained for the sixth time that month that "I just had to do it, Dad," that he needed to be alone for a little while before he could talk to his son without making them both feel more overwhelmed.

After regaining emotional control, do something kind and soothing for yourself.

Whatever you decide to do, it will be done under your balanced emotional control rather than under the sway of negative emotions, and that will undoubtedly feel better to you. As I have stressed before, it is very important that you practice these skills in noncrisis situations first. Practice emotional mindfulness when you're annoyed at a waiter, or when you see a sad story in the newspaper or on TV. Use the ordinary moments in life to practice these skills.

CHANGING WHAT YOU FEEL IN THE MOMENT: OPPOSITE ACTION TO CURRENT EMOTION

Imagine that you just noticed that your child has a new cut on her wrist. You thought she was in distress an hour or so ago, but when you asked her if she was okay and if she needed any help, she said everything was "fine." In this situation you would most likely feel a combination of worry, sadness, and anger: worry that your child is still resorting to self-injury, sad that she's unhappy, and anger that when you offered help, she denied there was a problem. As the day wears on, you find that these painful feelings keep circulating through your mind, making it difficult to stay focused at work and impossible to take pleasure in the good things that happen during the day. You are stuck in the feelings generated hours ago. Clearly you need a way to change your current emotional state.

The skill set that will help you in these situations is *opposite action to current emotion*. It means you are deciding to change the way you feel. If what you're feeling seems appropriate to the situation, though, you may not want to change it. For example, if you have experienced the loss of a loved one, you want to stay with the sad feelings as part of the grieving process.

Simply put, opposite action to current emotion requires you to choose an activity opposite to what your current emotion is pushing you toward. For example, if you're like most people, when you're feeling depressed and lethargic your body tells you get in bed and pull the covers up over your head. You have the impulse to get out of life and just lie still. The opposite action would be to deliberately and with conviction get involved in an activity. While this is certainly easier said than done, with some effort you can achieve great results. Staying with this example, you might decide to take a brisk walk or go to the gym.

> *Your goal is to change the way you're feeling. Want to crawl into bed? Take a brisk walk instead. Feel like screaming and pounding the wall? How about some soothing music instead?*

All emotions have a corresponding *action potential*. Anger tends to make us move toward attack, for example, while fear makes us withdraw, and shame makes us want to hide. Once you recognize an emotion's action potential, the trick is to pick an activity that is its direct opposite. For example, you come home and find blood-stained tissues in the bathroom again, and your child has left a note saying he's gone to a friend's house and won't be back for several hours. After calling him and checking in, it wouldn't be too surprising if one of the emotions you felt was anger. You think about calling him back and insisting that he come home, or you think about how you're really going to let him have it when he gets back. But wait! You notice (mindfully) that you are just cooking your anger, and in fact you want to change the way you feel. You decide to do something nice either for yourself or for someone else. So instead of giving in to the action of the angry emotion, you prepare your favorite dinner for the family.

Opposite action to current emotion is a very effective skill but one that is difficult to master. In order to optimize your chances, I believe there are three critical things to keep in mind. First, understand that this skill is about acknowledging what you feel in the moment. It's not about denying what you're feeling or judging what you're experiencing—it's only about accepting how things are in this moment. Second, be sure to accurately label the emotion you want to change and its corresponding action potential. You can do this by using your emotional mindfulness skill. You must know what you're feeling in order to take the opposite behavioral action. Third, you have to totally commit to doing this skill. You will not reap the benefits if you participate in a half-hearted fashion. Opposite action to current emotion requires that you throw yourself into the activity 100%. The following are some guidelines for opposite action to the particular emotions of sadness, anger, fear, shame, and guilt.

Feeling	Opposite action
Sadness	Physical movement
Anger	Do something nice for yourself or someone else
Fear	Face it
Shame	Face it
Guilt	Either repair it or tolerate it

Opposite Action to Sadness: Physical Movement

As I suggested earlier, sadness and depression seem to drain us of our energy. Often it feels as if we just don't have what it takes to do the simplest of tasks.

All we want to do is lie down and rest. We are preoccupied with dark thoughts, and it feels as if our lives will never get better. The action potential for depression is to stay still. If, however, you decide that you want to shake the blues, then choose an activity that requires physical movement. You don't have to run a marathon. Try a quick-paced walk, turn up the music and dance, or go to the gym. I think you will find that your mood will change as you get involved in the activity.

Samantha felt that she could hardly get out of bed when she awoke, and instantly remembered the new scabs she'd seen on her daughter's arms the evening before. As she remembered, an intense wave of sadness came over her and, with it, a powerful urge to pull the covers up and go back to sleep. She felt extremely fatigued. She knew she had to get up to go to work, but her body was telling her to stay in bed. She recalled the skill of opposite action to current emotion and decided to try it. She turned on some music and began to stretch.

Opposite Action to Anger: Do Something Nice

When we're angry we want to strike out and go on the attack. Sometimes this is just what the situation requires, but often attacking will only make the situation worse. We feel stuck in our anger and begin to ruminate on the unfairness of the situation. We imagine what we would like to do or say to the person with whom we are angry. We cook our anger until it takes over our mind and ruins our day. If you're angry and can take an appropriate action to improve the situation, then by all means do so. For example, if you feel slighted by your spouse and think that a discussion will resolve things, then do it. In those instances where there isn't any effective action you can take, however, rather than cook your anger into a spicy ragout, try opposite action.

In the case of anger, opposite action would be doing something kind for yourself or for another person. Send someone flowers or make your spouse a special dinner or inquire after an old friend. Trust me: getting involved in acts of kindness will help dissipate your angry feelings.

Opposite Action to Fear: Face It

When we're frightened or worried about something, we have a tendency to avoid those situations that are likely to elicit this emotion. For example, parents who have a child who is engaged in self-harm often become fearful of confronting him or her about something out of the worry that it will cause an argument that will lead to self-harming behavior. When we give in to fear and avoid situations that require action, we now have two problems instead of one: the original problem plus the sense of diminished self-regard that we typically feel when we know we're avoiding something because of our worry.

So if fear is making you avoid something that really needs to be addressed and you are troubled by a sense of diminished self-esteem, approach the problem head on. Do what you're afraid to do. Again, I suggest that you practice this skill on the small worries first. If you're afraid of telling a bossy friend that you have to cancel a dinner engagement, for instance, take a deep breath and just do it. Let yourself have the experience of knowing what it feels like to approach and master fearful situations—I guarantee it will work wonders on building your confidence to tackle the harder issues.

Opposite Action to Shame: Expose Yourself to It

Shame is such an awful emotion. Shame makes us want to disappear and hide. Parents who have a child who engages in self-harm frequently experience this emotion in situations where they have to explain something about their child's status to a friend or relative or to the school or another institution. People work very hard to avoid the experience of shame. Sometimes when parents avoid shame they are unwittingly cutting off their noses to spite their faces—that is, they may be depriving themselves of the much needed help and support available from friends, relatives, and institutions.

The trick is to make the best assessment you can about who in your world can be trusted with this very sensitive information and speak with them. You want to avoid sharing information with people who are going to induce shame—that is, those who are likely to negatively judge you or your kid. Once you have figured out whom you can trust, then I suggest that you deliberately speak with these folks about your situation. When you do this, expect that shame will rise to the surface and, as it does, just notice the experience without avoiding it.

The psychological principle at work here is known as *exposure*. It turns out that when we are racked with shame, exposing ourselves to the experience without judging ourselves or avoiding the experience will diminish the intensity of the shame. The same principle is at work if we listen to a favorite song over and over again—after a while it loses its charm for us. The more you do this exercise, the less shame will be a factor in your life.

Opposite Action to Guilt: Repair or Tolerate It

What parent doesn't feel some guilt about his or her parenting? A certain amount of guilt just seems to be an occupational hazard, but being overrun by guilty feelings will leave you feeling awful about yourself and put a black cloud over your life. Here are some ways you can manage your guilt.

There are two central questions to ask yourself that will help you figure out whether your guilt is warranted or unwarranted. It's an important differentiation to make because warranted guilt requires you to make a repair and an apology, while unwarranted guilt requires you to tolerate your distress without the repair and apology.

1. Are you *responsible* for having done something, either unwittingly or intentionally, that has been harmful to your child, or does your guilt arise from some judgment about yourself that is less reality-based? Here is an example of what I mean. On Sunday night your son asks if you can pick him up after school on Tuesday rather than his having to take the bus. He tells you that he wants to get to his friend's house as early as he can because all his friends are getting together to play a new video game. You agree and tell him that you will be there. That is the last time you and he discuss the arrangement. Tuesday comes and you are swamped at work. Your agreement to pick him up just falls out of your head. Around 3:30 the phone rings: it's your son asking where you are. In all likelihood you are going to feel a little guilty about having forgotten to pick him up. In this situation it would make perfect sense that you would feel guilt.

2. Have your actions violated your ethics or values? Molly's 14-year-old daughter has come in way past curfew over the last several weekends without any good explanation. An important value in their family is that members keep their word about the commitments they make, and that if they can't keep a commitment they will let people know about it in a timely manner. Furthermore, Molly is pretty certain that some drinking may have occurred on these occasions. The last time she was late, Molly put her on notice that the next infringement would result in a grounding for the following two weekends. The girl acknowledges that she understands the consequences for being late. The next Friday night she comes home 2 hours late with no phone call. She understands that she'll be grounded.

Several days later, however, she informs Molly that next weekend her former best friend, a girl who moved away years ago, is coming back to town for just one night. She pleads with Molly to cut her some slack, but Molly holds her ground in what turns out to be a very upsetting interchange, leaving the girl sobbing in her room for hours. That's when the guilt starts bubbling to the surface, pushing Molly to reconsider the limit she set. Her guilt is getting the best of her and she wonders whether sticking to her guns is the right choice. Is Molly's guilt warranted or unwarranted?

Most of the situations we encounter as parents are not clear-cut cases of warranted or unwarranted guilt, and this one's no exception. Let's take the example apart. I think everyone would agree that Molly was well within her parental rights to set the limit and that the conditions for grounding are fair. In fact, I think we would say that she would have been remiss in her duties had she not set the limit she did. Furthermore, at the time the limit was set, the daughter seemed to understand and accept the consequences for her lateness. So far so good, but now it gets tricky.

While it is true that her daughter is hurt by the limit because she can't see her friend, I don't think we can hold Molly *responsible* for her daughter's hurt feelings, nor can we say that Molly has done something that is at variance with her own values or ethics. The daughter is responsible for her response to the punishment; her mother may feel understanding but shouldn't feel guilty. Consequently, the guilt that Mom feels is unwarranted, and she should act opposite to the emotion and not apologize and/or undo the consequences. Her daughter will not be able to see her old friend.

In short, warranted guilt requires a repair and an apology, and unwarranted guilt requires that we tolerate our distress and stick to our guns. Opposite action to current emotion is a powerful skill that, when effectively used, will help turn down the temperature on negative emotions and increase moments of calmness, happiness, and pleasure. What parent wouldn't want more of that?

TAKE CARE OF YOURSELF

I really don't want to sound like your guilty conscience, but it's just a fact that managing your life with balanced sleep, healthy eating, reasonable exercise, and avoiding excessive use of alcohol and other substances reduces your susceptibility to the negative emotions. For example, in times of stress our bodies need good nutrition to manage the extra workload. All too often in such times, we just don't have the energy or feel we don't have the time to eat right. We skip meals, eat more fast food than usual, and/or soothe ourselves with rich desserts. While all of this is understandable and I certainly would not encourage you to move to a Spartan diet—after all, having some treats in your life is a good thing—I ask you to be mindful of your body's nutritional requirements. You will feel better and have more resilience to get through the hard times if you do.

Living somewhat off the mark can limit your capacity to fully experience moments of happiness too. Just think how tough it is to enjoy your day when you are sleep-deprived or hung over. Often when our lives become more stressful—and living with a child who engages in deliberate self-harm certainly is among the most stressful—we often resort to coping strategies that may work in the moment but leave us more depleted in the long run. Having that extra drink or glass of wine are examples of strategies that may promise short-term relief but generally work against us in the overall scheme of things. The stress associated with a child who has emotional troubles can cause you to lose sight of the healthy things you need to do for yourself as you throw yourself into the process of helping and getting help for your child. Exercise, healthy eating, and activities you find fulfilling are often casualties of the process. You may sacrifice doing the things you enjoy in order to be more available to your child. When I meet with parents who have a child who is self-harming, I routinely ask them what they are doing to lower the stress level in their lives. If they tell me that they've given up almost everything they used to enjoy, I encourage them to get back into those activities that make life a little more worth living.

SIGNS THAT YOU NEED TO TAKE BETTER CARE OF YOURSELF

1. Are you eating more fast food or junk food because it just seems easier or quicker?
2. Are you feeling tired all the time?
3. Are you feeling pressured and stressed by things or events that you ordinarily have taken in stride?
4. Are you more irritable?
5. Do you have the sense that there is no time for you anymore?

RELATIONSHIP MAINTENANCE

As the song goes, "You always hurt the one you love," or, in some cases, the one you used to love. Relationships are always tested in times of stress, and parenting relationships are no exception. At the very time when the parenting partnership is most in need of protection and maintenance, it often falls by the wayside when a child has emotional difficulties. All too frequently different parenting styles that have been overlooked in the past are now called into question as possible causes of or at least contributors to the child's self-injurious behavior. Long-standing difficulties in communication that were annoying at worst now become major points for concern. As the relationship worsens, the possibility that it could be a source of comfort goes down the drain. Parents feel wronged, alone with their worry, and angry. Keeping the parenting relationship alive, vital, and a source of comfort are of critical importance in helping you stay balanced.

Coming to a Meeting of the Minds

It seems to be a human tendency that when we are stressed, we fall into black-and-white thinking. If one parent is right, then the other parent must be wrong. Discussions can quickly deteriorate into heated battles over whose position is true and why the other person's is false. Feelings are hurt, and anger and frustration take the day. The relationship, no longer a source of support, becomes yet another problem to be solved. One way to avoid this awful situation is to work at maintaining a dialectical discussion (see Chapter 4 for a review). The following pointers will help you avoid those dead-end discussions:

1. As hard as it may be to believe, you don't have the corner on the market on truth, nor does your partner.
2. Ask yourself, Do I want to be right or do I want to be effective?
3. Work at finding at least the grain of truth in your partner's point of view without giving up on the grain in yours.
4. Look for what each of you is leaving out of the picture.
5. When the discussion gets back on track, validate your partner and yourself. Validation at this point might just accomplish two things. First, it may smooth the way for the discussion to continue in a reasonable manner, and second, it may reinforce more effective communication.

Repairing the Relationship

In order for you to use your relationship, whether it is with your primary parenting partner or not, as a source of comfort, you have to know how to make a repair when things have gone south. I can almost guarantee you that being skilled at this will maximize the support and comfort you get to reduce the stress in your life. The good news is that you don't have to learn a new skill; the GIVE skill I outlined in the previous chapter is the one to reach for.

Often the hardest part of making a repair is overcoming your aversion to making the first move. If you ask yourself questions like "Why is it always me who has to apologize first?" or "I wouldn't have said the things I did if she hadn't started in with me" may be 110% correct—but, again, the essential question is: Do you want to be right or do you want to be effective? "Effective" in this case means working at repairing the relationship so you can get more of what you need. The choice is up to you. I urge you to find the willingness to move in the direction of doing the things that will help you get the comfort, support, and pleasurable moments that you need.

Keeping the Relationship Strong through Action

I'm going to end the chapter with a section on maintaining your primary adult relationship. When that relationship is running smoothly, you are in a better position to weather the hard times with your kid. Relationships work best when time is set aside just for the couple. Keeping the couple strong and vital goes a long way toward preventing parental burnout and helps you to create times of comfort, pleasure, and support.

Keeping your primary relationship strong takes deliberate action. While spontaneity is wonderful—and I encourage you to find those special moments when things just seem to happen—don't let your relationship slide for lack of planning. Make time for going out to dinner, seeing a movie, or, if possible, going away for a weekend. Whatever happens for our children, there will most likely come a time when they will leave home. When that time comes it will be just you and your partner, so protecting the relationship now is a very wise investment in your future. Remember that this is not a dress rehearsal, but time in your life that you are not going to get back. Taking care of your relationship is taking care of yourself. Your child will be better off for your efforts.

> Whatever happens for your children, there will most likely come a time when they will leave home. When that time comes it will be just you and your partner, so protecting the relationship now is a wise investment in your future.

In this chapter I've focused on the immediate triangle of you, your partner, and your child. In the final chapter, I'll help you navigate your way in the wider sphere of the other children in the family, as well as your child's friends and school.

9

how to speak with siblings, friends, and the school about your child's troubles

Getting a grip on your child's problem by understanding where it came from and how it can be treated is a giant step. Self-harm is a difficult enough problem for you, your child, and the therapist. But you also need to negotiate your way in the wider world during the time your child is being treated. In this chapter I'll share my advice on the complicated and delicate matters of communicating with your child's siblings, friends, and school.

SIBLINGS

"Mommy, I know something's wrong with Samantha. I heard you and Daddy talking last night. Is she going to be okay? Why does she hurt herself? Doesn't she like herself? Is she going to have to go to the hospital?" asked 8-year-old Tommy.

"Samantha is having some worries now, and Dad and I are making sure she gets the help she needs," his mom replied. "I'm glad you asked, because we know you have noticed how upset she gets sometimes, and how your dad and I have been worried about her. Are you worried about your sister?"

"Yes! I get kind of scared when everybody gets so upset and worried," Tommy said. "Sometimes it seems like you guys just forget about me and only think about Sam."

Another sibling of a teen who self-harms, 16-year-old Bill, had this to say about his sister: "I think she's just a drama queen looking for attention! You and Mom are just being idiots and don't see that. You know she doesn't even try to stop, and all you guys do is give her the attention she wants. Plus you send her to that shrink, who isn't doing anything and is costing a fortune."

"Slow down here, Bill," his dad responded. "I know it seems like she's doing this for attention, but we don't think that's the whole story. We know this makes you angry. Your sister is pretty unhappy right now. Please do me a favor and just open your mind to other possibilities about why she cuts herself."

"Like what? That she enjoys the pain or that it makes her feel cool?" Bill replied sarcastically.

"Actually, I didn't have those in mind. I know how upsetting this is to you, and I think more information would help. Your mom and I are concerned about how this is affecting you. If you can find a way to open your mind to your sister's seemingly crazy behavior, I can try to tell you about some other possibilities, and I think you'd feel better about how we're handling it," Dad replied.

A child who self-injures affects every other member of the family. If you have other children, it can be very hard not to allow the one who self-harms to become your primary focus. I encourage you to stay mindful of the other children's needs for your time and understanding. Knowing that your other sons or daughters are angry or jealous because one child is getting all the attention hurts. Naturally you don't want them to suffer, and you hope they could feel empathy toward the troubled sibling.

Let me make it clear that their reactions of anger and worry about whether they're going to get their own needs met are totally normal. They may even be angry with you for not being able to "fix" this problem quickly. In the following pages I offer some guidelines for how to deal with your other children so that they don't feel ignored.

Validate Siblings' Experience

The best tool to help you, once again, is validation. If you can validate how hard it must be for them and be nonjudgmental about their anger or other negative feelings, not only will it be easier for them to manage what's going on with their sibling but they'll also stay connected with you. Maintaining that connection will help them get what they need from you and be more resilient in the long run.

Drop Guilt and Turn to Empathy

Let me say something about guilt. Every parent has it, whether or not his or her kids are struggling. We have it because we all have limitations. There isn't one of us who parents perfectly at all times. Good parenting actually involves being aware of our limitations so that we don't push ourselves further than we can go. When you have a child who is not doing well, worry about whether you have been a good parent can expand to huge proportions. Add other children who may have to sacrifice some of your time and energy to their troubled sibling and the situation is ripe for guilt. It's hard to accept that you can't do it all, but of course there will be times when you can't. Be aware of your guilt and respond to your children with empathy rather than trying to make it up to them with gifts or material things.

Stay Involved in Your Other Kids' Lives

Of course having a child who self-injures is going to demand more of your time, but make sure to find ways to be part of the other kids' school and extracurricular activities. On those occasions when you have to miss an event because of an appointment or because you're just worn out and need time for yourself, be sure to offer the other child an alternative time when you can be together. Think about involving other adults in their lives to add to their support system. While no one can take your place, having another caring adult available who is aware of your child's problems can make all the difference when you and the child's other parent are stressed and temporarily distracted. Consider informing teachers or guidance counselors that the family is under stress so that school personnel can be on the lookout for problems and available to step in to offer more support should they need it.

Talking about Their Sibling's Self-Harm

The other kids in the family frequently don't know if, or how, they should address the feeling that they're getting less from you, or how to ask questions or give voice to their worries. If you decide to keep your teenager's deliberate self-harm a secret from the other children in the family in the hopes that it will protect them from undue stress or safeguard the injuring child's privacy, you may unwittingly create a number of additional problems. Kids are very perceptive. They probably know that something's going on, but the climate of secrecy will deter them from getting information that might help them manage their concerns. So the secrecy only results in depriving them of adult help, leaving them to struggle with their anxieties alone. In addition, being aware of a secret may communicate to the other kids that something's going on that is so awful as to be unspeakable. Consequently, the secret, rather than protecting them, may create more worry than is warranted.

How much the other kids in the family are affected depends on a number of variables, including their ages, the kind of relationship they have with one another, and their resiliency. Sometimes the other kids let you know about their feelings, and sometimes they remain silent. Knowing how to explain to the other children in the family about deliberate self-harm and how you as parents are getting the child the help he or she needs, and inviting the siblings to express whatever concerns they may have will reduce the tension in the family and help you all function in a healthier way. The following three factors are critical in helping you to establish guidelines that will steer you through these tricky waters.

1. Before you speak to the other kids in the family, you and your troubled adolescent must have a clear understanding about what information is going to be shared. Respect the self-injuring child's need for privacy, but at the same time address the needs of the other children in the family. Negotiate what information is going to be shared and with whom, and whether the adolescent is going to be part of the discussion. What is nonnegotiable is *whether* information is going to be disclosed or not. Notice below how Samantha's dad is validating but firm. See how he does not back down in the face of Samantha's rising emotions. Balancing validation with clarity and calm firmness is the path you seek.

2. What you say to the sibling depends on his or her age. Kids in elementary school need a more global but clear version of what's going on, while children in middle and high school can probably tolerate a more factual version of their sibling's behavior. Notice how Samantha's father is very clear about how he and his wife are managing the situation and how he remains responsive to his son's worries without burdening him with too much information. The most important principles with younger children are (a) to be honest without giving them more information than they can handle, and (b) to convey the sense that while things are troubling, you are in charge and capable of managing the situation.

Adolescents may know other kids who self-injure and may subscribe to some common misconceptions about the behavior, or they may harbor critical judgments about what kinds of people resort to self-injury. Often adolescents, especially boys, use anger and contempt to distance themselves from their worry and concern for their sibling. On the other hand, they may have some real capacity for empathy and concern that might translate into support for their self-injuring sibling.

Early adolescents may need a slightly different approach than kids who are 16 and older. Kids in this age group (middle school) vary, sometimes moment to moment, between being adolescent and being more like a younger child. Consequently, how much information you share with them depends on your assessment of their level of maturity. Children who are closer in maturity to younger children need the information in more general terms, while the more mature kids can use more detailed information that might include a discussion about the function of self-injury and how their sibling is getting the help he or she requires. In either case, adolescents, like younger children, need to be made to feel that there is room for their questions and their concerns.

3. Be careful in gauging the capacity and resiliency of the children to manage the information about their sibling. Some things you need to take into consideration are how much stress the child is currently under, whether he or she is an emotionally sensitive person who is likely to be overwhelmed by too much troubling information, and whether he or she has other outlets that may help in modulating these worries. Taking these factors into consideration will make you better able to think through how and what you want to say to the other children in the family. The following lists will help you assess how much stress your child may be experiencing currently.

CHECKLIST IN APPROACHING YOUR ELEMENTARY SCHOOL CHILD

1. Is your child more silent and withdrawn than usual?
2. Does your child seem clingy and needy?
3. Does your child have school or behavioral problems?
4. Is your child having trouble sleeping or falling asleep?

CHECKLIST FOR OTHER TEENS IN THE FAMILY

1. Does he or she seem more withdrawn than usual?
2. Is your teen staying away from home more than is customary?
3. Does he or she seem irritable with you?
4. Has there been an increase in behavioral or school difficulties?

"Samantha, your mom and I need to speak with you about how we're going to talk with Tommy about the problems you're having," said Samantha's dad.

"I don't want you to say anything to him. It's none of his business, and anyway he will blab things all over the neighborhood!" Samantha angrily replied.

"Your Mom and I want to protect your privacy *and* help Tommy with any worries or questions he may have," Dad answered.

"I don't want him to know!" Samantha countered quickly.

"While we want to be sensitive to what you want, Tommy, let Mom know that he knows something is going on for you and that he's confused and worried," Dad replied.

"I have all these problems, and now you guys are making it worse. Why can't you think about how I feel for once?!" Samantha said with anger and sadness rising in her voice.

"The fact is, we're all worried and concerned. Tommy needs some taking care of too. Do you want to be part of the discussion? Then you can tell him how important your privacy is to you," Dad replied in a calm but firm manner.

"All right, I guess. I don't like this one bit, but I didn't know he was worried. Yeah, let's talk with him together," Samantha suggested.

Finding a way to help the other children in the family understand what's happening with their sibling will go a long way toward easing your mind and helping you feel a little less overwhelmed. The trick is to find the middle path between not burdening the children and respecting their capacity to manage a difficult situation. Keeping these guidelines in mind will help you come to the right decision for your family members. Now let's talk about dealing with people outside the immediate family circle.

EXTENDED FAMILY AND FRIENDS

What, and how much, should you tell extended family members and friends about your child who self-injures? It's a difficult issue. Let's start by figuring out why you're talking to them about this delicate family matter.

What Is the Goal of Sharing the Information?

The best way to think about sharing information with extended family and friends is to get clear about your goals for doing so. As with speaking with siblings, it's important that before you share any information you let your teenager know with whom, what, and why you're sharing this very sensitive information about her. So take a little time and ask yourself a couple of questions that will help you get clear about your goals.

First ask yourself, What is my objective in sharing this information? Am I looking for a source of support? Do I expect the person or people with whom I'm going to share this information to be understanding and supportive or judgmental and critical? Are these people likely to be supportive to me but critical and judgmental of my child? For example, a friend might convey support for you by blaming your kid for putting you under so much stress. Conversely, he or she might be supportive of your teen but blame you for the child's difficulties.

Can You Protect Your Teen's Privacy Adequately?

Second, can I trust them not to share this information with other family members or friends who may not be supportive? Or do I need to provide just enough information about the situation to protect our family's privacy?

For example, your child has cuts on her arms and she and you feel that it could be awkward to go to the family reunion at the lake this year. Her brother and sister have been looking forward to the reunion for months and would be terribly disappointed if they couldn't go. The extended family knows that your daughter has been having some kind of emotional troubles, but they're not aware that she self-injures.

What are you going to do? You and your daughter might be more willing to be forthcoming if you were pretty sure that the response from others was going to be warm, supportive, and understanding. If that were the case, disclosing the information beforehand might be the right thing to do—it would make it easier for your daughter to attend the reunion, and you might feel taken care of by your relatives. On the other hand, if sharing information were likely to make the situation worse, then the best course of action might be to give very limited information about your daughter and see if you could make arrangements for her to do something else during the reunion. That way her brother and sister would not be penalized because of her troubles and you would not lose out on going to the family gathering. Let me explain how I'm using the phrase "limited information."

Is Lying Ever a Good Idea?

You're in a tough situation, and there may be some circumstances that would make you want to lie about the troubles at home. For example, if you know that someone holds the belief that there's no such thing as a psychological problem and that therapy is a bunch of hooey, being totally honest with that person about what's going on with your child is most likely to lead to an awkward conversation at best. If you think that all you're going to get from this person is judgment and grief, but you do need to provide some explanation, lying might seem like a reasonable strategy.

I believe, however, that lying brings with it a whole host of unforeseen problems. It compromises our sense of integrity, and that erodes our self-esteem. For most people the usual emotional response to telling a lie is feeling guilty, and nobody enjoys that emotion. Furthermore, when we're caught in a lie, we most often feel ashamed. And it almost goes without saying that lying complicates our interpersonal relationships. If the self-injuring teen becomes aware of the lie, it could give her the message that what she's doing is so horrible that it must be covered at all costs. Don't you have enough to deal with already with this troubled child?

My advice: Avoid lying whenever possible. That doesn't mean you have to disclose everything about the situation at home, just enough to be effective in achieving your goals. When you hide the full story, it's generally better to stick with some partial truths rather than fabricating untruths.

So what should you say? Most people know at least a little about depression from news stories or from people they know who have suffered with it. Because kids who self-injure are often depressed, it's not such a stretch to focus on that aspect of their troubles. It lets someone know the general realm of the problem (mental health) without violating your teen's privacy. You can talk also about "difficulties with coping" and "problems with self-esteem," both of which, again, tell a partial truth without revealing too much.

Of course, these partial truths will work only in those situations where the teen's scars are not visible. Most kids are reluctant to allow other people to see their wounds. There are, however, a minority of kids who do want people to see them, either as a communication about their distress or as an expression of anger or rebellion. I would suggest that you have a discussion with your child about the impact of her scars on other people and why you believe discretion is advised. If she insists on displaying her scars, then I would let her know that it will be her responsibility to explain to people what's going on. Also let her know that you're going to be open with people and give your version of events.

If she continues to show her scars, you will be in a position of having to be honest with people and to educate them as best you can, but you should also suggest that they speak directly with your daughter. Be mindful of using your distress tolerance skills, as this is potentially a very stressful situation. You always have the option of not allowing the child to see these people if that seems the most prudent strategy.

Accepting Others' Limitations

No matter how careful and skillful you are, there are some harsh realities you'll need to manage. There will be people who distance themselves from you or your child because they're afraid of what he does. People can find self-injury frightening and deeply disturbing. You can't educate everyone, especially while you're also trying to take care of yourself and your family. If your child loses friends, or her friend's parents won't allow contact because they learn of the self-injury, be validating to the loss. Over time these natural consequences may help channel some of your child's energy into change and recovery.

What to Say to Those You Trust

You need to hold on to the relationships that will be most sustaining for you, and that means trusting your instincts about whom you can talk to openly and honestly. Most parents find it comforting to have a select group of people with whom they can be honest. Talking with too many people in an attempt to get support will usually leave you feeling exposed and vulnerable. You'll probably have a few people in your life with whom you will want to share this problem, and in order to elicit support, you might have to demystify it.

Here are some guidelines for those few close friends and extended family members you'll want to share this with:

- Explain that self-injury is most often a way for a person to cope with overwhelming emotions.
- Counter any misconceptions they may have about self-harm, such as it being a suicidal gesture.
- Be clear about what you need in terms of support—that is, request that they listen without giving advice, or ask specifically for help with problem solving.
- If you're concerned that sharing this information will change their opinion of you or your child, be open and talk it through with them.

THE SCHOOL

It's not uncommon for kids who self-injure to have problems in school. These difficulties can be of a social nature, an academic nature, or both. Kids who self-injure are often mood-dependent. Consequently, when they're feeling sad, angry, or overwhelmed, they may have great difficulty paying attention in the classroom or completing homework assignments. Caught in a downward spiral of missed assignments and poor grades, their attitude toward school deteriorates. As soon as you become aware that your child is falling into this pattern, it's time to access additional school services.

In addition, school forms the basis of a teenager's social life. It is the primary place where kids develop and learn how to manage interpersonal relationships. Often, when a child begins to self-harm, rather than being supportive, other children may withdraw from the friendship. This can also have a negative effect on the child's attitude toward school.

It's important that you find ways to make the school environment as positive an experience as it can be. This may require working with the school to make an individualized education plan, or IEP. The key is to respond quickly when you notice that school is becoming a problem, either academically or socially, for your child.

How and When to Have the Discussion

School personnel may very well be the first adults to find out about your child's self-harm. Another student might get concerned and alert them, or a teacher may notice the wounds. Once this happens, the school is required to take some kind of action. Schools are very worried about the copycat effect that self-injury sometimes generates in a community of adolescents.

In my experience, schools respond in a variety of ways, from simply notifying you and asking you to take your child to the pediatrician to requiring the child to take a medical leave until the behavior is resolved. In any case it is likely that you will be in an ongoing dialogue with the school. In situations where the school knows about the self-injury, your best course of action is to be forthcoming with information about the treatment you're getting for your child and the progress he or she is making. Always maintain a good working relationship with the school, as you may need to access their services in the future. Depending on how sensitive and understanding your school personnel are and how your child feels about bringing the school more into the know, it can be a good idea for the school counselor to have periodic updates from your kid's treatment team. The bottom line is that when the school knows about your kid's behavior, being straightforward with the facts is the best course of action.

In those instances where the child's deliberate self-harming behavior comes to light out of the purview of the school, parents are confronted with a very different situation. The question then becomes, Do you tell the school or not? Making this decision is similar to deciding whether and how to tell friends and extended family. The first step is to get clear about your objective in disclosing the information and then make some Pros and Cons Charts about the various options.

For example, if your child is going to be out of school for a couple of weeks, you are going to have to say something to the school. If your objective were to let the school know so that the teachers could provide missing schoolwork for your child, but you're concerned that the school may be less than sensitive about the issue of self-injury, then you would evoke the "limited information" guideline. You might say something about serious personal problems that your child is experiencing that are being actively addressed and that you'll let the school know when your child will return. On the other hand, if you believe that the school would be more supportive and understanding if they had a fuller picture of the circumstances, then you should be more explicit about the problem.

As you can see, sharing the information will require you to make a judgment call. Work hard at noticing and tolerating any shame, embarrassment, or guilt you feel that may compromise your abilities to make a decision in the best interest of your child. This will help ensure that you make the right decision and won't second-guess your course of action.

Finding the Right Placement

The high school experience is as much about learning how to socialize, to be part of a community, and to develop appropriate romantic relationships as it is about getting an academic education. Learning how to negotiate these rather complex matters is part of the task of any adolescent. Consequently, whenever possible, the educational setting should mirror the one that the child would have been in had she not developed these difficulties. If the child was headed toward a vocational or arts high school, you should try as best you can to make that match. At this point you are probably saying, "This sounds great, but how do I make it happen?" Good question.

Only a few of us will have the means to pay privately for the educational setting that is best for our child. Most of us will have to rely on the special educational services provided by our local school system. School systems are required to provide special educational services to children who are having difficulties being educated due to physical or psychological reasons. The laws around special education mandate schools to educate children in the least restrictive setting. What that means is that they're obligated to find the most "normal" school that your child can manage. That can translate into a mainstream setting with some extra counseling, at one end of the spectrum, to a therapeutic boarding school, at the other end.

Parents can access these services by requesting in writing that the school undertake an evaluation of the child's needs. Public school systems are *obligated* to do this. At the end of the evaluation, if it's determined that your child qualifies for service, the school will develop an IEP. The IEP is a binding contract that the parents and school sign. If you don't agree with the services spelled out in the IEP, do not sign it! This is where knowing how to talk with the school gets critical.

Special Programs

The first thing you need to keep in mind is that the laws are written in your favor so, with the right strategy, odds are you are going to get pretty close to what your child needs. So don't start with a "big stick" approach. You are your child's advocate, while the school has other concerns: they need not only to match your child with the right services but also to consider available program spaces and financial constraints. While that's not your problem, being sensitive to it is an important part of being effective.

Second, do your homework. Educate yourself about all the different programs the school district offers. Then make an assessment about the one you think is best suited for your child and which ones might be reasonable alternatives if there's no space available.

Finally, if you and the school can't seem to get on the same page, several courses of action are open to you. First, you can work with an educational advocate who will help you negotiate with the school system. Some advocates provide services for free, and others work on a fee-for-service basis. You can probably get a list of advocates from the school system, from the yellow pages, or off the Internet.

Or, you can hire a lawyer who specializes in helping parents get the help they need for their children. The American Bar Association (ABA) website (*www.abanet.org*) contains links to referral services in each state, many of which will help you identify lawyers with experience in special education and disability law. In my experience this step almost always makes the process adversarial, and should be used only as a last resort.

The take-home message is that with knowledge and perseverance, you will most likely come very close to getting what your child needs. One way to get started in locating educational advocates and/or lawyers to help you in this process is use the Internet and search for educational advocates. This search will produce any number of sites that will guide you in locating some-one in your area.

More Than 4 Years

One of the biggest stumbling blocks for parents and kids is thinking about high school in a time frame other than the customary 4 years. I really want to help you get past this view. While there are some downsides to your child's not graduating with her class, these are usually minor in comparison with ei-ther not getting the treatment she needs or being in an educational setting that stresses her beyond what she can reasonably do.

Not graduating with your class is a short-term problem. I can't tell you the number of kids I have seen who did not graduate with their class, received the help they needed, and in a few short years were right back up to speed. Take the long view on this issue and don't succumb to the pressure of having to complete high school in 4 years.

Looking Ahead

Now that you've read this book, I hope you have the understanding and the tools to help your child and yourself. I have no doubt that practicing the skills that I have outlined will, over time, help you to manage your own feelings and to be more useful to your child. Remember to practice validation before problem solving; use your mindfulness skills to help you see things as they are, without judgment or being pushed around by your emotions; and count off the distress tolerance skills to help you through times of crisis. In your darkest, most painful moments, remember that everything changes—the moment you're in will change too. You now know that while there is no quick fix and that eventually your child can get the problem under control, deepening self-knowledge and learning important lifelong skills along the way.

One last reminder: Always keep the long view—this is not a sprint, but a long-distance run. I believe that with new tools, perseverance, and, whenever possible, a little humor, you will come out of this with a better appreciation for your kid's strengths, more confidence in yourself, and a better relationship with your teenager. You can do this!

APPENDIX A

effectiveness of adolescent intensive dialectical behavior therapy program

Two Brattle Center's (TBC) Adolescent Intensive Dialectical Behavioral Therapy Program is designed to improve the psychological, behavioral, and social functioning of adolescents experiencing emotional dysregulation and/or self-injurious or self-defeating behaviors. TBC is committed to providing evidence-based treatment and to monitoring clinical change over the course of treatment to ensure that clients are improving in desired ways. Toward this end, we conduct bi weekly assessments with all clients in this program and provide the results to clinicians and families so that they can track and ensure desired change over the course of treatment. We measure changes in psychological distress, symptoms of depression and borderline personality disorder (BPD), emotion regulation skills, self-injurious thoughts and behaviors, and overall functioning within the family, socially, and at work.

Presented below is a summary of the change observed for a consecutive series of 42 clients treated in the adolescent DBT program during 2005–2006. The purpose of this brief document is to provide objective information about the average amount of change experienced by adolescents and families participating in our program (individual results vary).

OVERALL PSYCHOLOGICAL SYMPTOMS

Over the course of treatment, adolescents reported a significant decrease in the overall experience of psychological distress (depression, anxiety, anger, etc.), as measured by their report on the Brief Symptom Inventory (BSI), a commonly used psychological measure of psychological symptoms. Scores changed from an average of 90.77 before

From Hollander, M., Wheelis, J., Photos, V. I., & Nock, M. K. (2005, November). Intensive outpatient models of adult and adolescent DBT: Development and initial evaluation. In J. H. Rathus & M. K. Nock (Chairs), *Bridging the lab and clinic: Advances in the measurement and training of emotion regulation, mindfulness, and interpersonal skills*. Symposium conducted at the annual convention of the Association for Behavioral and Cognitive Therapies, Washington, DC. Reprinted by permission.

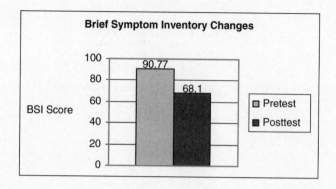

treatment to 68.10 after treatment, moving from the very high end of the clinical range to a level that falls within the normative range for outpatient clients. This amount of change in only a 4-week period compares very favorably to that observed in other treatments.

DEPRESSION

Over the course of treatment, adolescents reported a significant decrease in the experience of depressive symptoms, as measured by the Beck Depression Inventory, a commonly-used measure of depressive symptoms. Scores changed from an average of 29.23 before treatment (which represents the "Severely Depressed" range) to 20.76 at posttreatment (which represents the "Mildly to Moderately Depressed" range). Here too this amount of change in only a 4-week period compares very favorably to changes observed in other outpatient treatments.

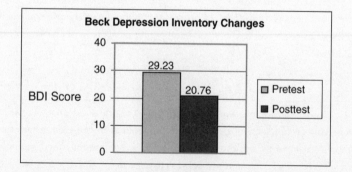

SYMPTOMS OF BORDERLINE PERSONALITY DISORDER

Adolescents in our program endorse an average of 6.8 symptoms of BPD at the start of treatment (five out of nine are needed to meet diagnostic criteria for a BPD diagnosis), and this decreases to 4.8 symptoms at the end of our 4-week program.

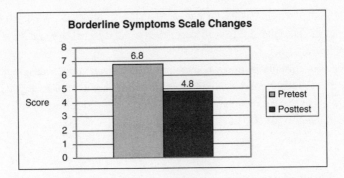

SELF-INJURIOUS THOUGHTS AND BEHAVIORS

Adolescents in our program report a decrease in the experience of thoughts and behaviors of nonsuicidal self-injury (cutting, burning, etc.) as well as suicidal thoughts and attempts. The figure shows the average number of each behavior reported in the 2 weeks before treatment compared to the last 2 weeks of treatment.

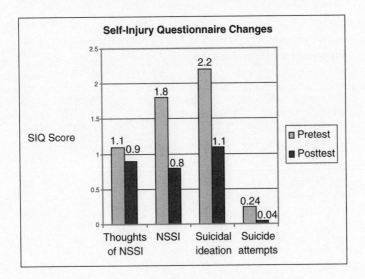

Overall, adolescents participating in this program report significant improvement in each of these domains, as well as in the development of emotion regulation skills and functioning at home, socially, and at work (additional data available upon request). Of course, changes in each area are not absolute, and most adolescents continue to experience some psychological and behavior problems at the end of this 4-week treatment—at which time a less intensive therapy schedule (typically 1–2 hours per week) often is recommended. However, the changes obtained during this 4-week period are substantial and are much larger than those reported in most other outpatient treatments.

We hope this information is helpful in providing data on the average amount of change that is to be expected in our program. We encourage you to ask additional questions about this treatment and its effectiveness, and we are pleased to provide further information to the fullest extent possible.

APPENDIX B

intensive treatment programs

In this appendix I want to familiarize you with treatment programs that run the gamut from 24/7 programs in an inpatient setting to those that meet multiple times a week for a few hours.

INPATIENT PROGRAMS

In this day of managed care, most inpatient hospital stays are relatively short, from a couple of days to a week or two. The task of an inpatient stay is crisis stabilization, medication adjustment, and aftercare assessment and planning.

Inpatient hospital units are the most restrictive level of psychiatric care. The doors are locked, and the child's freedom is significantly curtailed. While each unit has its own protocol for treatment, generally the child is seen once a day by a psychiatrist who will be assessing and possibly altering the psychopharmacological regimen. There are nursing staff members available for check-ins throughout the day. Parents usually meet with a social worker, who is most likely meeting with your child too. The social worker has the major responsibility for developing and coordinating the child's after care plans. If the treatment team has questions about diagnosis, they may call in a psychologist to administer some psychological testing.

Today psychological testing is not routinely part of the treatment protocol, so don't expect it to be done unless you advocate for it. Short-term hospital stays can be very useful in helping to develop a more effective outpatient program, in changing medications, and sometimes just providing a time out for you and your child. This kind of inpatient hospitalization, however, in all likelihood will not be long enough, nor geared directly enough, to resolve deliberate self-harming behavior.

ACUTE SHORT-TERM RESIDENTIAL UNITS

Short-term residential units are often used as a step-down from an inpatient setting or as an alternative to inpatient care. These units are accessed when the clinicians in charge of admission determine that the child can be managed in a slightly less restrictive setting. Unfortunately, these units are not as widely available as inpatient programs, so there may not be one in your area.

The typical length of stay on these units ranges from a week to a month. By and large these units are slightly less restrictive than inpatient settings. Kids have a bit more freedom for passes and privileges, but still have a very structured treatment schedule. Typically there are fewer psychiatrists and nurses than on an inpatient unit, but often more social workers and psychologists. The clinical task of the short-term residential unit is similar to that of an inpatient unit, but the longer stay can sometimes build a stronger foundation for the outpatient work to come.

DAY HOSPITALS AND INTENSIVE OUTPATIENT PROGRAMS

Day hospitals and intensive outpatient programs (IOPs) are nonresidential and less restrictive than inpatient and acute residential programs, but still provide a very structured therapeutic environment. Length of stay is quite variable, ranging from a few days to several months or more. At this level of care the patient, the clinicians, the parents, and the managed care people (if they are involved) often have some flexibility as to how many days a week the child will attend the program, how many hours a day, and how long a stay it will be.

Some day hospitals and IOPs are generic programs, which means they accept adolescents who have a wide range of behavioral and psychiatric issues. Others are more focused on a narrow range of problems and provide a specific treatment approach. For example, the IOP that I oversee is a DBT-focused program primarily for kids who self-injure or engage in other types of self-harming or self-defeating behaviors.

Assuming that the adolescent has a chance to stay for several weeks or more in an IOP or day hospital, some invaluable therapy work can get started. In addition, the longer time frame allows for medications to be reviewed and changed as necessary. Furthermore, the longer stay often makes parental guidance work and/or family therapy a much more viable option.

A downside of these programs is a direct outgrowth of their upside: longer stays and multiple meetings per week make the transition back to school or work complicated. Everyone who is connected to the child's treatment needs to think hard about the clinical benefits and liabilities of such a treatment choice.

LONG-TERM PROGRAMS

Long-Term Residential Treatment Programs—When All Else Has Failed

Marnie and her parents requested a meeting with me to discuss her lack of progress in therapy. Marnie was a 15-year-old girl who had been depressed, suicidal, and self-injuring since she was 12. Recently her parents had become concerned because Marnie was lying about her whereabouts, had taken up with an older group of kids who were known to use hard drugs, and had run away from home for several days at a time. They reported that her school attendance was declining, along with her grades. Marnie's parents told me that she had been hospitalized about eight times, had had multiple therapists, including in family therapy, and had been in a DBT program. The parents were exhausted and on the brink of despair. Every effort they had made had resulted in a dead end. No therapist or program had been able to contain her dangerous behavior or elicit even a modicum of collaboration in therapy. As you will see, I was no exception.

"So, Marnie, what is your understanding about why your parents wanted this meeting?" I asked.

"I don't know. Why don't you ask them? Do I look like a mind reader?" she shot back.

"I don't know, let me see. No, you don't look like a mind reader, but you do seem to be pretty angry. What's up with that?" I wondered.

"I don't talk to morons," Marnie replied, and she got up and left my office.

Unfortunately there are situations that require an adolescent to be sent for long-term residential care. When the child and her family have availed themselves of all the local resources but the situation just continues to worsen, this may be the only other option. For parents and children alike, it's an awful moment. The idea of your adolescent child being gone for months at a time for treatment may make you feel like failures, and guilty ones at that. Plus, in spite of all the trouble and heartache they've caused, it turns out you'll miss them like crazy! For the kids, being away from their home and friends can feel like the end of the world.

As painful as these moments are, they are sometimes the new beginning that kids and parents desperately need. In a somewhat arbitrary way, I am defining long-term programs as 18 weeks to several years. These programs always have some kind of school component (the exception might be some wilderness programs, which I will describe next). In fact, these kinds of programs run the gamut from school-based settings with clinical services to intensive clinical programs with a school component. These programs break down into two categories: those funded with public money and those funded with private money. Sometimes the publicly funded programs accept private funding, and occasionally a privately funded program will accept public dollars. As you can see, this gets complicated. For this and many other treatment programs, it can be useful to hire an educational consultant to help you think through all your options. Educational consultants can be accessed through the web. Often these professionals visit programs several times a year, and therefore are in a good position to make a match between your child's needs and a program.

Whenever possible, plan a visit to the program yourself, or at least speak directly to the admission staff. Many programs have a list of parents who would be willing to speak with you about their experience with the program. Remember, however, that these are likely to be the parents who had a good experience, not the ones with major disappointments. By the same token, brochures and websites offer limited useful information. I have never read a brochure for anything that didn't say its organization was the best at what it was providing!

Wilderness Programs

Sometimes when an adolescent is struggling, it's a good idea to shake up his routine. Wilderness programs do just that. The essence of these programs is twofold. First, the idea is to take the child out of his or her comfort zone and create an environment in which group members have to trust and rely on one another. Kids learn just how strong and resilient they can be when they only have the barest of creature comforts available to them. Second, within this Spartan existence the adolescents' usual defensive and ineffective coping strategies break down, opening the possibility for new and more effective strategies to develop. The length of stay at a wilderness program can vary from a couple of weeks to several months. Similarly, the degree of physical hardship runs the gamut from an Outward Bound–style experience to that of a summer camp.

Wilderness programs can become the first step toward helping your child regain some confidence and hope. In my experience, however, they need to be followed by an ongoing therapy program. When this doesn't happen, the gains made at wilderness program tend to vanish quickly. I strongly recommend if you are considering these kinds of programs that you work in conjunction with an educational consultant to find the program that best matches your child's needs.

Long-Term Residential Therapeutic Programs and Schools

Sometimes for kids like Marnie, when all else has failed, parents need to consider long-term residential programs. This is always a tough decision for parents to make. Sending your child away from home is always a loss, and parents should expect to feel some combination of relief and sadness.

There is a wide variety of long-term programs available for adolescents. Some are funded through public state agencies and others are privately funded. These are no easy options, though: the privately funded programs are very expensive (think college tuition, plus room and board), and those funded by public agencies generally have long waiting lists. The majority of privately funded programs are located in the southern and western parts of the country and are best accessed with the help of an educational consultant.

The privately funded long-term residential programs form a continuum from those that are highly restrictive with very structured behavioral and clinical programming to those that are more like boarding schools with clinical services. There are programs that emphasize outdoor activities and those that concentrate on the arts.

For parents who are going to access publicly funded programs, the good news is that these programs are generally closer to home; the bad news is that they usually have a very long waiting list and treat a broad range of children. Consequently, adolescents who are involved in self-harming behaviors may be in the same program with kids who have very different types and severity of problems. It is very important that you ascertain what kinds of troubles are being treated in the program and whether a differentiated approach is taken depending on the child's diagnosis.

Often publicly funded programs use a cost-share model between the department of education and the department of social services and/or department of mental health. It is sometimes hard to figure out the system. If you're having trouble navigating the system, most states have educational advocates who work with parents and kids to make sure the child is getting the right kind of services. You can obtain a list of educational advocates through the special education department at your child's school.

Nonresidential Long-Term Placements: Therapeutic Day Schools

Lakisha had been attending a high-powered independent school until the school nurse noticed that she had been self-injuring. Following school policy, the nurse notified the school counselor and the dean of students, and a meeting was held with Lakisha and her parents. At that meeting the school determined that Lakisha needed to take a medical leave and would be allowed to return to the school the following year if her self-injurious behavior had been adequately treated.

Lakisha was glad to hear that she could return to school, but what was she to do in the meantime? Before attending her independent school, she'd been at a large public high school and found the size and overall commotion a trigger for her self-harm. What now?

Lakisha should consider a therapeutic day school. These are publicly funded schools that typically have small classroom settings, teachers who are sensitive to their students' mental health needs, and clinicians on staff. Generally these schools have the required academic accreditations to keep students up to date with credits and required courses. Therapeutic day schools are often ideal next steps for kids who are leaving more restrictive programs (long- or short-term settings) and who might lose ground if they returned to a mainstream high school environment.

Like the longer term programs, these schools offer a range of educational and clinical services. Some schools are geared toward those who are college bound; others aren't. Some schools have a hefty clinical emphasis; others don't. When thinking about therapeutic schools, make sure you know about the academic as well as the clinical programming and about the kinds of children who attend the school. For example, does the school generally educate kids with severe behavior disorders or is it more geared toward adolescents with depression, anxiety, and self-injurious behavior? The idea, as always, is to find the best fit for your child. Your teen's therapist or an educational advocate can be a good resources to help you find that fit.

RESOURCES

websites related
to self-injury

The scores of websites that focus on self-injury fall into two main categories: (1) websites designed by professionals to assist self-injurers, and (2) websites created by self-injurers intended to offer peer support. Brief descriptions of several of the more prominent websites of both types are provided below. This review is meant to be representative, not exhaustive.

WEBSITES DESIGNED
BY MENTAL HEALTH PROFESSIONALS

Self-Injury and Related Issues (SIARI)
www.siari.co.uk

The SIARI website is the creation of Jan Sutton, who is based in the United Kingdom. She is the author of *Healing the Hurt Within: Understand and Relieve the Suffering Behind Self-Destructive Behaviour* (How To Books, 1999) and several other books.

The multifaceted website, with its many links, provides many helpful suggestions regarding coping skills and alternatives to self-injury, a self-assessment questionnaire for self-injurers, and first aid information. It also offers information for family and friends, references to many publications regarding self-injury, and a bookstore. An interesting and unusual feature is that the website offers an online support group for *professionals* who work with self-injurers. I am not aware of any other website that has this feature.

There is a well-designed *moderated* message board for self-injurers, with guidelines for participants about the dangers of posting triggering information and a request to label it as triggering to forewarn others.

The website presents a "cycle of self-injury" that includes the steps of (1) mental agony, (2) emotional engulfment, (3) panic stations, (4) action stations, (5) feel better, and (6) grief reaction. In all likelihood, Sutton's cycle does not apply to all self-injurers but primarily to trauma survivors and those who tend to dissociate. The SIARI website provides an article by Sutton regarding the link between self-injury, dissociation, and trauma. Although some of the content of the SIARI site may not be relevant for self-injurers from the general population, the suggestions regarding coping skills and alternatives to self-injury are relevant for all.

S.A.F.E. Alternatives
www.selfinjury.com

The S.A.F.E. Alternatives website is the creation of Karen Conterio and Wendy Lader, authors of *Bodily Harm* (1998). This website offers concise material about self-injury, a brief summary about the components of successful treatment, a bibliography, and links to purchase Conterio and Lader's book and video. The website also provides a link for admission to their inpatient unit at Linden Oaks Hospital at Edward, in Naperville, Illinois. This program is the only inpatient unit devoted exclusively to the treatment of self-injury in the United States. Optimally, the length of stay for this program is 30 days.

Conterio and Lader also operate the national information line—800-DON'T-CUT—which has been an invaluable resource for self-injurers for many years. This line receives about 16,000 calls per year and their e-mail address (wladersafe@aol.com) another 5,000 contacts (Wendy Lader, personal communication, 2004). That Conterio personally responds to the phone calls and Lader to the e-mails indicates their heroic level of commitment to help self-injurers.

American Self-Harm Information Clearinghouse
www.selfinjury.org

This website is the creation of Deb Martinson, the author of the notable "Bill of Rights for People Who Self-Harm." It is a strong statement of affirmation for self-injurers that clients and therapists should read.

The website carries Favazza's endorsement and offers a brief description of the reasons for self-injury, a discussion of myths regarding self-injury, self-help suggestions, and several links.

There Is No Shame Here
www.palace.net/~llama/psych/injury.html

This is another website by Deb Martinson. It is a complex site that offers information about causes of self-injury, self-help, diagnoses, treatment, and information for families and friends. There is a lengthy list of references and many links. The site offers a monitored message or web board for self-injurers that carefully addresses the issue of triggering content.

The site provides *many* suggestions for replacement behaviors, although some are questionable, such as slashing a plastic bottle or heavy piece of cardboard. Such aggressive modes place a weapon in the hands of self-injurers and may make self-harm more likely. The website takes great pains to be accepting, supportive, and nonjudgmental toward self-injurers.

Self-Injury
www.mirror-mirror.org/selfinj.htm

This simple one-page website presents some basic information about self-injury and concentrates on presenting a long, useful list of alternatives.

WEBSITES CREATED BY SELF-INJURERS OFFERING PEER SUPPORT

LifeSIGNS: Self-Injury Guidance and Network Support
www.lifesigns.org.uk

This website is run by a set of directors, "some of whom self-injure, some have beaten self-injury, and some have never self-injured" (quotation from the home page of the site). (I have classified this site under the self-injurer-generated category because some of the directors have considerable experience with self-injury.)

This comprehensive site is very professional in appearance. It offers extensive information about self-injury and suggestions for eliminating the behavior. It has a chat room with clearly articulated rules about avoiding triggering content. The authors of the site have written several pamphlets on self-injury, designed for schools and universities, that are available through the site. A monthly electronic newsletter is offered to members. Many links are provided. The site also offers a "Self-Injury Charter," which is similar in some ways to Deb Martinson's Bill of Rights. This appears to be among the best of the peer-generated sites in terms of offering positive, supportive, nontriggering, solution-focused content.

RecoverYourLife.com
www.recoveryourlife.com

This website (formerly RuinYourLife.com) offers a complex combination of benefits and risks. This site is "dedicated to exploring 'self-destruction' in all its forms."

There is no doubt that websites of this type help some self-injurers feel that they are not alone and that their problem can be discussed with others. This multifaceted site offers self-help suggestions, a first aid section (which may be triggering because of its level of detail), and a gift shop selling RYL journals, mouse pads, mugs, teddy bears, and clothing.

Of concern are the poetry and artwork. Some of the art includes graphic color photos of wounds and drawings of lacerations, wounds, and blood. One drawing depicts a person who has died by hanging. In my opinion, the risks that this site takes in terms of triggering cannot be justified. I did consider not drawing attention to it in this appendix, but the site does come up on the first page or two of a Google search of "self-injury."

Self-Injury: A Struggle
www.self-injury.net

This website is said to have been generated by a young adult self-injurer named Gabrielle. She states she has been self-injuring for 7 years. Although attractively designed, some of the content is alarming—such as the section titled "Gallery of Pain." This category contains artwork that depicts razor blades, wounds, blood, and the like. There is also poetry describing acts of self-injury and at least one short story that culminates in a completed suicide. The site has sections on famous self-injurers and a memorial section for self-injurers who have died. The categories on stopping self-injury, helping family and friends, and finding resources seem less developed than the more negative content areas. There is a message board offered, but I could not find rules or even a statement pertaining to concerns about triggering content.

This is the type of site that provides some support for young self-injurers, but also contains a great deal of triggering material that could do harm. Aspects of this website run the risk of normalizing and even *glamorizing* self-injury. The content is weighted heavily in the direction of describing and depicting self-injury rather than solving the problem of self-injury.

Self-Injury Support
www.sisupport.org

This rather simple peer-generated website is based in California. The mission of the site is "to offer a positive and productive self-injury support site providing alternatives to self-injury, referrals, support groups, affirmations and interactive opportunities" (from the homepage). This site was developed in response to sites such as the two described immediately above. The Self-Injury Support website states, "Much to our dismay we have discovered that many [self-injury websites] . . . are 'triggering' and not exactly the type of material we wanted to read about when we were struggling ourselves, usually late at night, with thoughts of self-injury. So, we have decided to focus on positive information regarding self-injury and hope that you will find our site to be both educational and supportive in a positive and reassuring manner to help those in need."

Consistent with these goals, the site emphasizes understanding self-injury and how to recover. There are lists of references and programs that serve self-injurers. There is no chat room.

index

about the author

Michael Hollander, PhD, a recognized expert in the treatment of self-injury, has worked with adolescents and their families for more than 30 years. He maintains a private practice in psychotherapy, conducts dialectical behavior therapy with adolescents at McLean Hospital in Belmont, Massachusetts, and serves on the psychiatry teaching faculty of Massachusetts General Hospital and Harvard Medical School.